T
5/02

SURVIVING MADNESS

SURVIVING MADNESS

A Therapist's Own Story

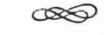

BETTY BERZON

B
BERZON
2002

The University of Wisconsin Press

The University of Wisconsin Press
1930 Monroe Street
Madison, Wisconsin 53711

www.wisc.edu/wisconsinpress/

3 Henrietta Street
London WC2E 8LU, England

1   3   5   4   2

Printed in the United States of America

Library of Congress Cataloging-in-Publication Data
Berzon, Betty.
Surviving madness: a therapist's own story/
Betty Berzon.
pp.   cm. — (Living out)
ISBN 0-299-17620-7 (cloth)
1. Berzon, Betty. 2. Lesbians—United States—Biography.
3. Lesbian psychotherapists—United States—Biography.
I. Title. II. Series.
HQ75.4.B49 A3   2002
305.48'9664—dc21   2001005833

This book is dedicated:

To the late Paul Monette, who taught me to dig deeper and write better and not be afraid of my anger.

To the late James Leo Herlihy, who said the magic words, "Are you crazy? Write the book!"

And, as always, to the very much alive Teresa DeCrescenzo, without whose love and encouragement I'd still be thinking about writing a book someday.

⧉ Acknowledgments

Jed Mattes, for agenting all those books and for being my friend.

Trude Berzon, for being such a good stepmother.

My sister, Dr. Stephanie Miller, and the Miller family, for being such loving caretakers of mother and grandmother.

Shirley Schloss-Wool, Sidney Wool, and Sandy and Jerry Wool, for being cousins you *want* to share your life with (Abbe and Danny, too).

Dr. Peggy Kemeny and Dr. Michael Van Scoy-Mosher, for saving my life (Michelle, too).

Michelangelo Signorile and Gabriel Rotello, for being courageous writers and good friends.

David Gerstner, Mitchell Ivers, and Mark Swersky, for being a great audience and listening to my stories.

Michael Lassell, for his editorial help.

Raphael Kadushin, Joan Larkin, and David Bergman, for having confidence in this book.

And the late greats, Minnie and Maxie, and the presently wonderful Molly and Mandy, for keeping me company every day as I wrote.

Some of the names of people in this book have been changed or omitted, either to protect their privacy or to preserve the illusion of their innocence.

SURVIVING MADNESS

Come with me to a psychiatric hospital on the outskirts of Los Angeles. See in the bed a young girl, wrists and ankles tied to the bed rails, eyes staring through the barred window, silent testimony to the mind-blanking effect of depression.

I am that young girl, being protected from myself, restrained against the vein-slashing suicide attempt that brought me here. I am twenty-two years old and I am certain that my life is over.

Then see the girl one year later, same hospital. She wears a white coat and is a member of the electroshock team, gently holding a patient's legs as he convulses in response to the jolt of electricity being shot through his brain. She works in the hospital now, recovery in progress, a new career underway.

I am *that* girl, too, and the one who studies psychology and becomes a therapist and sits here now telling the story of how it all came to be. It is a story that reflects the joy of achievement and the fun of defying convention at long last to claim an authentic identity, one that does not have to be okay with absolutely everybody.

Today I am the woman, the seasoned therapist, the writer who passes on what I know about the need to explore illusions, the elation of insight, and the power that love and sex, experienced as one, can have on redefining identity.

Come with me to trace the interconnections that weave the splendid fabric of identity. The process of psychotherapy gave me incredible strength for this endeavor. Through it I learned not to be afraid of my emerging self but to welcome change, to accept desire, to allow passion. This is a tale of sanity in the world making sanity in the individual more possible, where the patient becomes the doctor, and madness becomes the teacher of healing.

I was brought into this world by two bewildered teenagers who were as unprepared for their passage into parenthood as they had been inattentive to ways to prevent it. As if having a baby were not terrifying enough, I was born with a gaping hole where my palate should have been. For the first nine months of my life I had to be fed every few hours with a medicine dropper, head held back to ensure the flow of nourishment down my throat rather than out my nose. It was not a good beginning for any of us.

Fortunately for me, my parents lived at the time with my maternal grandmother and my mother's four sisters and one brother. My aunts took turns feeding me, including ten-year-old Esther, who would climb into my crib and pretend she was feeding her little baby doll.

At five months I was taken to visit Dr. Vilroy P. Blair, a renowned plastic surgeon who practiced in St. Louis where we lived. By some miracle, my young impoverished parents had connected with this famous man, who declared he would operate to close my palate when I reached nine months, leaving four more months of water-torture feedings.

I shudder when I think of the fragile infant that I was on that operating table, but Dr. Blair obviously knew what he was up to because the surgery was a success. The worst part of it, I'm told, was my mother's reaction when she first saw the bloody sutures hanging out of my mouth. She fainted dead away and refused to visit me again until the sutures had been removed.

The cost of that surgery in 1928 was $100, including pre- and postoperative care. I still have the bill. The cost of the trauma suffered by my mother when she saw those bloody sutures was much greater, setting the stage for an abiding fear in me of my effect on her that would play out over my entire childhood.

When I was nearly two we moved to our own apartment. I'm sure that I missed the attention of all those aunts, but liberated from the rigorous feeding routine and the worry of a sick child, my mother appeared to warm toward me.

In the summer my parents would take me on bicycle rides through the lush green acres of St. Louis's Forest Park. I rode in the handlebar basket of my father's bike, hugging my knees, feeling the breeze against my face. I remember those outings as though they occurred in slow motion, dreamlike, everyone happy, everything perfectly balanced, the world as it was meant to be.

Our family got through the Great Depression thanks to prostitution. My father was in the credit clothing business, going to his customers' houses to sell his merchandise and to collect the installment payments—$2 down and $1 a week. As a salesman he had the perfect combination of persuasiveness and charm. His handsome, dapper appearance included a serious mustache and an ever-present cigar, which made him look older than his years.

Prostitutes were his best customers. He'd make the rounds of the brothels that continued to prosper even as people stood in lines at the soup kitchens. Sometimes, on Sundays, he would take me with him as he made his "stops." I waited in the car while he disappeared into these mysterious establishments.

One Sunday I decided to rummage through the stacks of white cardboard boxes piled high on the back seat of the car. I was curious about the miniature dresses I found folded neatly under layers of tissue paper. They looked like little girls' dresses, but they were big enough for a grown person to wear. When my father returned to the car I asked him what these garments were. "Shut those boxes and mind your own business," he snapped.

That, of course, just aroused my curiosity more. I continued to work on the problem until I had occasion to ask my cousin, Sidney, a whole year older than I, what he knew about the dresses, for his father was in the same business.

"Teddies. They're teddies that the whores wear when they see their customers," he announced triumphantly.

"How do you know that?" I demanded.

"Boys just know certain things," he said.

I decided to leave it at that. Solving the mystery of the teddies was enough without delving into the vagaries of what boys knew that girls didn't.

In the winter of 1935, when I was seven years old, I awoke one morning unable to breathe. I ran into my parents' room, crying and gasping for air. The doctor was called and in minutes I was on my way to Jewish Hospital, a frantic trip that would be repeated many times for the next five years. In

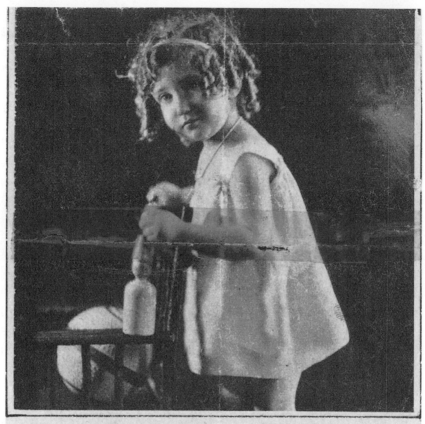

בעטטי בערזאָן, נעװינערין פון ערשטען פּרייז אין דעם קאָנטעסט פון •
שעהנע קינדער אױף דעם „פּאָרװערטס" באַלל אין סט. לואי.

Chosen as the prettiest child at the St. Louis Jewish Forward Ball, 1932.

the hospital I was placed inside a huge oxygen tent that covered half the bed. I was almost lost to sight in its vast interior. Inside all that plastic I lay quietly waiting to die, terrified but resigned.

I didn't die. A week later I was breathing normally again. A few months later I was back in the tent, another asthma attack, another mad dash to the hospital. Jewish Hospital became my second home, actually a kind of haven from my fear that both my parents, but especially my mother, would tire of my illness and the problems it caused and abandon me, just run away and be done with me. The nurses at Jewish Hospital were always kind and affectionate and welcoming. Eventually, I began to wish that I lived in the hospital all the time. I almost did.

When I was ten my parents brought home a red-faced, squalling little bundle who, I was told, was my new sister, Stephanie. I was not happy with this, worried that I would get even less attention from my mother. That worry was well founded because Stephanie turned out to be the easy child I was not. She was pretty, healthy, and compliant. To add to the insult of her arrival, I sometimes had to take care of her. I was not the best caretaker, allowing my ambivalent feelings about her existence to be expressed physically in little jabs and shoves, nothing to leave any marks, of course. Many decades later she assured me I had done her no permanent damage.

Asthma seemed to be a mystery to the doctors in those days. They tried every treatment they knew before we moved on to what I thought of as exile. First my mother and I were sent to the California seashore where the fresh salt air was thought to be a remedy. Then we shipped out to the Arizona desert where the hot dry air was thought to be a remedy. All I knew was that I was falling behind with my little crowd of girlfriends in St. Louis and I might as well never go back. Magically, that was arranged.

Early in the morning of December 7, 1941, the Japanese bombed Pearl Harbor and the war was practically on our doorstep. For reasons I've never understood, my father decided that was the time to move us lock, stock, and barrel out of St. Louis to live in Tucson, Arizona.

I liked that move. Tucson meant starting over and getting away from the tight group of friends who by then had probably cast me out anyway. Everything about St. Louis felt tight to me. I was not happy in the middle-class Jewish ghetto where I had always lived. At a young age I was aware of the pressure to be like everyone around me, but something inside me rebelled against it.

The others in my crowd of six little girls seemed quite satisfied to blend their identities into one another's, taking their cues from a collective sense of self-importance. I had a lot of doubts about how important I was or whether I was okay as a person. I was shaky in my sense of myself, never as confident as all the rest seemed to be. I felt different but I had no idea why.

At fourteen I started dating boys. Maybe it was developing a life outside my family, or maybe it was the desert air after all, but something healing occurred then—my asthma disappeared completely.

War was my hobby. For years I had kept a scrapbook of newspaper clippings about the battles in Europe. When there was show and tell in school, I proudly brought my scrapbook. The teachers seemed disconcerted at this

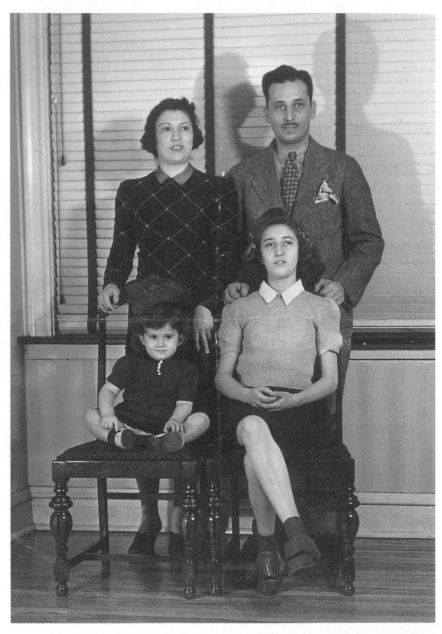

The whole family still living in St. Louis: mother, father, sister Stephanie, and an almost adolescent Betty.

interest of mine and the other students seemed uninterested. I didn't know why I had this strange preoccupation with war, but I also wondered why no one else seemed so fascinated. It was the most interesting thing happening in the world.

I went to every movie about combat. Star-crossed lovers and battlefront heroes were my romantic icons. I had not a clue, of course, of the blood-and-guts horror of war in real time. I only saw the glamour of it.

By 1942, World War II drew a little closer as shortages began to show up on the home front. Things we were accustomed to having plenty of were suddenly in short supply—butter, meat, coffee, and anything made of leather. Shoes were rationed, three pairs a year to each citizen. Each automobile owner in the country was allowed only four gallons of gas per week. Our government told us just to be glad we didn't have death raining down on us from the sky or battles being fought in our city streets.

There was no bloodshed on the city streets of Tucson, Arizona, but they were bustling with military. Davis-Monthan Air Base in Tucson was an embarkation point to overseas duty for Army Air Corps bomber crews. The young servicemen training to fly the big airplanes were not much older than I was—second lieutenants dashing in their crushed aviator caps, tan gabardine pants called "pinks," and perfect-fitting belted jackets. They looked like heroes and swaggered like tough guys, but I'm sure that underneath they were scared witless.

Many would never come back, and some would come back physically or emotionally wrecked. Their time in Tucson could be their last encounter with anything like a normal life.

I was sixteen when I started going out with flyers. They were so much more interesting than high school boys. The young flyers were grown up by virtue of what they were about to do. The hamburgers, milkshakes, and awkward groping of high school dates became rum and Coca Cola, dancing at the Blue Moon Ballroom, and a seduction routine involving military secrets.

I was slow-dancing to Glenn Miller with a young flyer at the Blue Moon. My date began to whisper in my ear, telling me that he feels like he is falling in love with me.

"Let's sit down," he said dreamily.

At the table, the young man grew solemn and took my hand. "I'm going to tell you something I'm not supposed to tell anyone. It's a military secret."

"A slip of the lip may sink a ship!" I heard in my head, the oft-broadcast

9

warning against talking about anything military. I said, "Why would you want to tell me a military secret?"

"Because I want to show you how much you mean to me."

That didn't make much sense because we'd only known each other a few days, but I was intrigued. He took out a pen and began painstakingly drawing on a cocktail napkin. When he finished he looked around to make sure no one was near enough to hear, then he leaned toward me and said, "Look."

"What is it?"

"It's the new, high-altitude, precision bomb sight that's just been installed in our B-17s. The Norden bomb sight. It's going to win the war for us. See, here's how it works," and there followed a technical explanation I didn't follow. When he finished, he picked up the napkin, dropped it into an ashtray, and set it on fire.

"You see, I've discovered that I really care about you, that's why I've told you this precious secret that I'm so excited about. Do you think we could go some place where we can be alone and get a little closer?"

"I don't think so."

"Please, this might be my last night here."

That in itself seemed like a good reason to decline. Patriotism aside, I stood my ground. He was disappointed, but after downing a few more rum and Cokes he seemed not to care anymore.

That young man shipped out and before long I was dating another flyer, then another, and another. Soon I could tell when the routine was coming as my date began fiddling with the cocktail napkin and looking very solemn. I sat through a couple more Norden bomb sights, complete with the ashtray fire, then always politely but firmly refused to go somewhere "to get a little closer." After a while I just stopped the routine as soon as it got started.

"I've heard it. I know all about the Norden bomb sight."

The young man would look startled, too embarrassed to ask where I'd heard about it. I wondered how often this routine actually worked or whether it was just one of those myths passed on in military bullshit sessions.

Between my scrapbook hobby, my immersion in war movies, and my patriotic dating of Air Corps flyers, I felt like I was fighting World War II on my own personal front. On August 6, 1945, the United States dropped the atomic bomb on Hiroshima, Japan. Three days later we dropped another atomic bomb on Nagasaki. On August 14, Japan surrendered. We won the war in the Pacific and introduced a device of mass destruction that has held the world hostage to its horror ever since.

In Europe, the Germans had already surrendered, Hitler was dead, Mussolini hung by his heels in a public square. Franklin Roosevelt, the only president I'd ever known, was gone. Everything was happening so fast. My world seemed to be turning upside down. There were no more flyboys to date. Tucson went back to being a quiet little desert town. My scrapbook was closed.

During the war years my father owned two bars and a restaurant, each mobbed every night with servicemen. My father loved the excitement of a crowded bar, people to schmooze, and new women to seduce. He was a habitual womanizer, often involved with a girlfriend and making no secret of it. My mother cried a river of tears.

The perpetual victim, my mother's outlet for her anger was me. She blamed me for everything bad that was happening in her life. At the time I didn't understand the dynamic of displacing her anger at him onto me. I simply felt very vulnerable to her. When she told me that I was the cause of her failing marriage, I internalized her feelings and made them my own. I hated my father for causing all this heartache, and I hated myself for being unable to relieve my mother's suffering or fix the situation.

How co-opted I was by my mother's dilemma, by the web these two emotional juveniles wove around me. I was trapped in their torment, powerless to help them or myself. She cried and he fled. I didn't know what to do. My own life seemed quite beside the point in this household.

There was so much pain at home I knew I had to find a way to escape it. My deliverance came through the Tucson Little Theater, a world that was distracting, seductive, and all-absorbing. The Tucson Little Theater was one of the best amateur community theaters in the country. I started out doing props, learned to do lighting, and graduated to stage managing. I loved being backstage where I could immerse myself in the cast-and-crew dramas that were sometimes as compelling as the theatrics onstage.

My life revolved around the theater. I was also studying acting, so I went from school to drama class, a quick dinner at my father's restaurant, and on to the evening's rehearsal or performance. I usually got home around midnight, but no one seemed to care about that except my French teacher because I often fell asleep in her 8 A.M. class.

It was about this time in my life that something was stirring in me that had me confused and concerned. I was having daydreams that were so preoccupying that I thought I was going crazy. These daydreams were all about women. There were romantic scenes in which I was Clark Gable or Errol Flynn sweeping some beauty off her feet, only the beauties were women I knew from school or from the theater, women I had developed intense feelings for though I didn't necessarily know them well.

My daydreams were not sexual per se, though I did think about holding these women, and I knew that was not what I was supposed to be thinking about. I liked dating boys, but I never had fantasies about them. It felt as though I were in love with women in a way that wasn't happening for me with boys. I didn't hear anyone else talking about such things, so I knew it was something I shouldn't talk about. I tried to shut off the thoughts, the intrusions into my thinking of this woman's face or that woman's body.

I was embarrassed by what was happening to me, hoping that no one could read my mind. The worst part was coping with what these fantasies meant. I'd heard of homosexuality, men loving men, women loving women, heard that it was a sickness, and I wondered if I had caught it. I had to know more about it.

The trip to the library was nerve-racking. I was afraid of what I would find. I looked all around before I pulled out the little wooden drawer marked "H." The books I took off the shelf told me that homosexuals were perverted, diseased, social outcasts, and pitiful creatures. That certainly was not me and never would be. Hurriedly replacing these volumes, I walked quickly out of the library, relieved to be outside breathing the fresh air. Whatever my feelings about women might be, they had nothing to do with the awful condition described in those books. I was sure of that. I was okay. I was normal.

Interview Eleanor Roosevelt? I was almost beside myself at the thought. As a reporter and feature writer for the Tucson High School *Cactus Chronicle*, I was always on the lookout for scoops, but this one would be monumental.

Just one year out of the White House after Franklin's death, Eleanor Roosevelt was a whirlwind of activity—a delegate to the United Nations, a syndicated columnist, on the lecture circuit, constantly visiting one corner of the world or another. I'd been a lifelong devotee of the Roosevelts. He was *my* president, elected when I was five years old, in office until I was almost finished with high school. Now, Mrs. Roosevelt was coming to Tucson to give a speech, and I decided I would somehow talk to her. Was I crazy to think I could get in to interview this legendary woman? "Well," I told myself, "they can't shoot me for trying," but I wasn't really at all sure they couldn't.

My big break came when I learned that Mrs. Roosevelt was speaking in the building sometimes used by the Tucson Little Theater. I knew that building intimately—where I could get in, where the star's dressing room was, where there was an open bathroom window I could climb through. Happily, I recruited a photographer to accompany me.

"Are you game for this?" I asked as we stood before the open window.

"Sure, why not, but what about the Secret Service?"

"She doesn't use them anymore. She convinced them to stay away after she learned to use and carry a gun." I'd read that somewhere and I dearly hoped I was right. We barely squeezed through the window and with hearts pounding proceeded to tiptoe into the hall. I jumped when I heard the voice.

"Well, hello there!"

We froze.

"Nice to see you again. Where are you headed?"

It was Howard Pyle, a famous war correspondent, soon to be governor of Arizona, whom I had recently interviewed. I took a deep breath.

"We have an appointment to interview Mrs. Roosevelt."

"Well, good for you. I just came from talking to her. I'll take you in and introduce you."

"Fine," I said, keeping my voice steady. "Lead the way."

I couldn't believe what was happening. Howard Pyle knocked on the door of the star's dressing room. A cheerful voice called out, "Come in."

Howard stuck his head through the open door. "Mrs. Roosevelt, I just ran into a young reporter I know from the local high school paper. She's here to interview you."

Mrs. Roosevelt smiled and waved us in. I moved slowly toward her and shook the hand she extended. Then I stood there, notebook in hand, and found that I was speechless. Seconds passed that seemed like hours.

"What would you like to ask me, my dear?" Mrs. Roosevelt inquired.

I pulled myself out of the dream. I was standing in front of Eleanor Roosevelt and she was talking to me. I don't know where the voice came from, but it began asking questions. "Where were you mostly educated?" the voice asked.

Mrs. Roosevelt answered that she was mostly educated in Europe, and in response to the next question, she described the ways in which European schools were different from those in America. "There is much more emphasis on learning languages because in Europe the countries are so close to one another." She also said she thought students of my generation were much more aware of contemporary world problems than they had been before.

"What do you remember as the most important thing that happened in your education?" I asked.

"I think the most treasured lesson I received during my schooling came from a teacher who had the remarkable ability to make one curious about things. She made you so interested in the subject that you wanted to go further and find out how and why it was so."

I scribbled furiously. As the interview progressed I became aware of feeling incredibly attended to by Mrs. Roosevelt, as though my questions were of the utmost importance. I understood later that this quality is the hallmark of a gifted politician, the ability to convey enormous interest in whatever is being said to them.

Several times during the interview we were interrupted by an assistant who, on first seeing us, looked alarmed. She knew we weren't scheduled, but Mrs. Roosevelt gave her an almost imperceptible nod. Not a word was said, but acceptance of our presence was established.

During these interruptions, I was able to observe Mrs. Roosevelt more closely. She wore a simple, long-sleeved black dress, topped by three strands of pearls, and at the V neck the Girl Scout pin so often seen in her photos. A corsage of gardenias was pinned to the left shoulder of her dress. In addition, there were two surprises—fire-engine red fingernails and a lacy black net over her short graying hair. I assumed the net was to keep her hair in place until she went onstage. But it never came off, and it was still there in the *Los Angeles Times* photo I saw of her a few days later, apparently a permanent hedge against a single hair escaping coiffed perfection.

I asked a final question. Mrs. Roosevelt responded with a long, thoughtful answer. I was momentarily distracted by the thought that should this building suddenly catch fire, Mrs. Roosevelt would undoubtedly continue to answer my question as she calmly led us all to safety.

One last request. Could we take a picture? She smiled graciously and motioned me to stand next to her chair. I did so and am forever recorded beside Eleanor Roosevelt in my tidy dark suit, clutching notebook and pencil, looking as though I had just done something of great moment, and indeed I had.

I sat in the audience afterward, listening intently to Mrs. Roosevelt's talk.

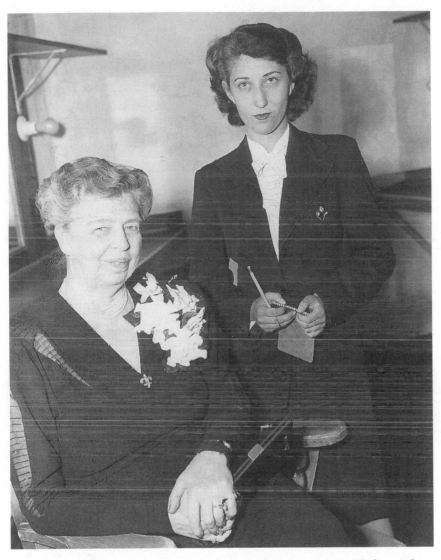

As a high school reporter scoring an exclusive backstage interview with former first lady Eleanor Roosevelt, on the lecture circuit two years after FDR's death.

She spoke of things I'd never given any thought to—the problems of young people whose countries had been the bloody battlefields of the war, who had not been able to go to school for five or six years, living precariously from day to day. "Ordinary standards of behavior do not suit them now. They have been living in an exciting world, a world where just outside the door death was imminent at all times. They have grown old very quickly.

It is difficult to find things that interest them, especially in their leisure time, for they must be taught that killing and stealing are not virtues in civilian life."

I felt deeply moved by her description of young people like me so scarred by living with death and destruction. I could hardly imagine what that must have been like. How shielded we were from those shattering experiences, so removed from the real horrors of war, so lucky, so safe. I felt as though I'd looked through a window at a world startlingly different from mine. I looked and was appalled that I'd ever thought there was anything romantic about war.

It took a long time for me to come down from the excitement of interviewing Eleanor Roosevelt, of spending twenty minutes in the company of this extraordinary woman. I had gone against my fear of being denied access to her and simply created access. I would remind myself of this success in future dilemmas about whether or not to attempt the impossible. I think she would have approved of the effect she had on me.

Four decades later, reading that Eleanor Roosevelt might have had lesbian relationships, I thought back to our encounter. I wondered how it would have been had we known each other's secret. Would I have felt better about my own homosexual thoughts if I had known this great woman shared that inclination? Or would I have thought less of her?

In a world where being gay no longer has to be a secret for a great many people, would Eleanor have revealed herself as a lesbian, and would she have been appalled or proud that all over the United States there are gay Eleanor Roosevelt Democratic Clubs? I would hope she'd be honored.

2

When I was a child in school in St. Louis, we were periodically administered something called the Stanford Achievement Test, through which I learned that there was a Stanford University. I had no idea where it was, but I was sure this Stanford was the fount of all knowledge, and I decided that I would some day go there to school. I held on to that fantasy all through junior high and high school. In 1946 my dream came true when I arrived on the Stanford campus, known as "the farm." It was no longer a fantasy.

Coming from a small family, the adjustment to dormitory living was not easy, but I learned to accommodate the relentless presence of others just as I learned the table etiquette and rules of social conduct that were a part of the informal curriculum of this rich-kids school. I heard classical music for the first time. When a round green thing was served at the dinner table, I watched closely to see what the others would do with it. I'd never heard of an artichoke. I listened carefully to the tales told by students whose families had taken them on trips all over the world. I absorbed information and soon began to imitate the speech patterns of those around me. If I couldn't be like them, at least I could sound like them. In so doing I camouflaged myself so I wouldn't stand out. Fitting in was the organizing principle of my life at the time.

My first year at Stanford there was just a smattering of males in the student body of three thousand. The war had recently ended, but demobilization was slow and only a few young men had begun to trickle onto college campuses. The following year would see an explosion of veterans flocking to universities under the GI Bill. That made the possibilities for dating much greater. Because I wanted to be like all the other girls, I enthusiastically chatted up the boys and joined in the endless rounds of discussions about who was dating whom, who I thought was cute, and who I wanted to go out with.

There were serious limitations on just how intimate a girl living in a dorm could be with her date. Males were not allowed inside the women's residence halls after curfew, making it necessary to say goodnight in the doorways, a favorite place for long, last-minute kisses. The private living quarters of girls' dorms were always off limits to male students.

It would have been mind-boggling to imagine that a few decades later men and women would be living on the *same floors* of university residence halls. The prudish restraints of campus life in the 1940s reinforced the mystique of sex, and the sexual prohibitions of the time probably only increased its allure. The sexual revolution was a long way off.

In my album of snapshot memories of those Stanford days there are the boyfriends. Bob was tall, bespectacled, and white-bread to his core. I think I was attracted to him because he seemed the epitome of upper-class breeding. He took me home to meet his parents in Pasadena. They were everything I had imagined they would be—reserved, refined, and stuffy. At dinner the subject of General Douglas MacArthur came up because he was very much in the news. I said I thought he was a pompous fool. Turned out he was the family's dearest friend. I was not invited back.

Next up was Tom, who introduced me not to his parents but to the great outdoors, which he loved. We hiked and camped and went fishing, all of which I cheerfully tolerated, but basically hated. Tom was different from anyone I'd ever gone out with, tough and tender; he had a journalist's curiosity and he dragged me to see things I'd never have known about if it weren't for him. Mercifully, he became editor of the *Stanford Daily* and was soon too busy to hike, fish, or camp. Our dating tapered off but we did remain friends, even after college.

Tom was followed by Ed, a fast-talking, aggressive New Yorker who had opinions about everything whether he knew what he was talking about or not. He was fascinating, but our relationship ended when I took a death-defying car ride with him and his friends to Los Angeles, during which they all sniffed from little white plastic tubes legitimately used to unclog cold-stuffed noses. They sniffed faster and faster, the car went faster and faster, and I hunkered down in the back seat scared out of my skull and waiting for the fiery crash that seemed inevitable. Incredibly, we made it there alive, but I took the train back to Palo Alto.

All three of my boyfriends became successful journalists, one an editor of *Business Week,* one the foreign editor of the *Los Angeles Times,* and one a network correspondent. I still find journalists the most intriguing people to be around. They are engaged in the world, well informed, and have a broader perspective on life than most people have.

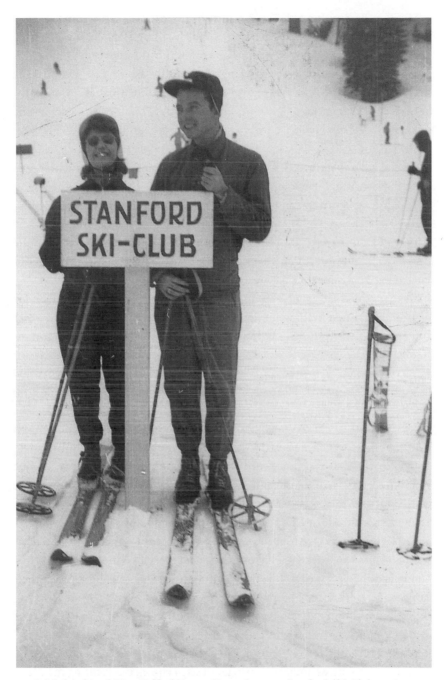

With boyfriend Tom Self, skiing at Yosemite on a Stanford Ski Club outing.

My own dream was to be a journalist or a writer. I took writing courses from the great Pulitzer Prize–winning author Wallace Stegner, who not only taught the nuts and bolts of writing but offered cautionary tales about life. I sat fascinated in his classes, wishing they would never end. One day he came into the classroom looking very grim. He contemplated the class for a few seconds, then in a flat voice announced: "This morning, an insane asylum in Asheville, North Carolina, burned to the ground and Zelda Fitzgerald with it."

Several people gasped. I waited for his comments. None came. He just made that stark statement and let it hang in the air. That *was* his comment, as if such were a fitting end to Zelda's aborted life journey and required no further elaboration. His Zelda announcement has stuck in my mind all these years, and I think of the simple impact of it when I am tempted to elaborate something endlessly, which I sometimes do to cover my insecurity about not having any impact at all.

Stegner was a tall handsome man with a craggy face. He had a flair for the dramatic, often holding his audience spellbound as he reeled out stories about the creative process. One such story he said contained an important lesson for us as writers. It was about a man who labored over a novel for seven years, then went into an emotional decline, and killed himself when the book was published. The man was Ross Lockridge; the book was *Raintree County*, which became a runaway bestseller and a blockbuster movie. The tragedy of Ross Lockridge was that he had been unable to separate himself from his work. When he lost his book to the public, he lost control of it. He could not call back one word. He was exposed to judgments, but he could not revise. "An author *is* his book," Lockridge wrote. Ross Lockridge was in his mid-thirties when he committed suicide.

The lesson in the story of Ross Lockridge for me was about the importance of keeping a certain professional distance from our own productions so that we may allow them a life of their own when it is time for that. When the job is done, let go of it. It is the lesson that parents must learn with their children. There is a time to allow separation so that everyone can move on to their own destiny. The lessons of writing often melded with the lessons of life in Wallace Stegner's teaching.

While I loved listening to Stegner in the classroom, I was discouraged by his reactions to my writing. He was relentlessly critical, discrediting my ideas, grading my writing low. I read those papers now and they look quite good to me considering that I was twenty years old when I wrote them. I began to feel he had something against me. Did I fall into some category that he resented? Had I annoyed him in some way? Perhaps it was because I was a sophomore and I'd talked my way into his senior writing class. Maybe I was too immature, maybe, maybe, maybe.

The Stanford campus is quiet on this sunny Sunday afternoon. Everyone is studying or at the Peanut Farm drinking beer. I am studying. The door to my room opens and Janet stands in the doorway, swaying slightly. Janet lives down the hall. She and I are friends, though we come from quite different backgrounds—hers old California money, Catholic, convent boarding schools, mine middle-class Jewish, midwestern, never away from home before.

Janet comes slowly into the room, a little drunk, a silly grin on her face. She sits on the arm of my chair and begins rubbing my neck. I'm uncomfortable.

"Are you all right?" I ask.

Without answering, Janet slides into my lap. She begins to nuzzle her face into my neck, kissing and giggling. I am afraid to move. I feel Janet's breathing against my body. I want to put my arms around her, but I also want to scream at her to get away.

"Janet, are you drunk? What have you been doing?"

Janet mumbles into my neck, "I was out with Richard, drinking. Listen, why don't we be lovers?"

She lifts her head and kisses me on the mouth, a long kiss I neither reject nor return. My head feels like it is going to explode; I have such a jumble of feelings—excitement, anxiety, anger. I feel assaulted.

"Janet," I shout. "What are you doing? What's happened to you?!"

"C'mon, let's be lovers. I've wanted to for a long time."

Panicking, I stand up and unceremoniously dump Janet off my lap. She just gets up, giggles, leans over, and kisses me again. I push her away. I'm terrified now.

"Oh, don't be so afraid," she says.

I take a deep breath. My voice is cold. "We can't be lovers. I don't even know what that means."

Janet rolls her eyes and says again, "Don't be so afraid."

My thoughts are spilling over one another. Is this a boarding-school game? What does she know about me? How can she be so casual? Why is she doing this? What is happening to me? In the sternest voice I can muster, I order Janet to leave my room.

"You're being ridiculous," she laughs.

"No, you're the one who is being ridiculous."

I'm sorry as soon as I say it, and Janet gives me a knowing look. She turns, walks to the dresser, and picks up my hairbrush. Smiling at me over her shoulder, she begins brushing her long auburn hair in drawn-out sensuous strokes. I watch, fixated, feeling out of my body, not daring to speak for fear of what might come out of my mouth.

After what seems like an eternity, she puts the brush down and moves toward the door. In the doorway she pauses. Staring at me, she nods as if agreeing with herself about something. She looks amused. The door closes behind her and she is gone.

I feel as though a great wave has just washed over me and left me standing. I want to shout, "Come back!" but it is only a silent scream. I am shaking. I feel very alone.

Janet and I never speak after that. I am too embarrassed to look at her. When the new quarter begins, I move to another dormitory, but it doesn't help. I don't want to think about Janet, but when I try to study, her face comes into focus, crowding out everything else. I'm doing poorly in school. I wonder if I'm going crazy. I daydream about that Sunday, Janet sitting in my lap, but I make it come out differently. She stays with me and I hold her and kiss her. I feel the excitement of her close to me. I want us to stay that way forever. I think I am terribly sick.

Over the next few weeks, I feel more and more disoriented. I am consumed with thoughts about what I have become. Is this what I have been hiding from myself, refusing to allow into my consciousness until Janet kicked the door open? I don't want to go through that door, but I am so drawn—so repulsed, yet so drawn. I have to find out, but not with Janet. I don't trust her. She changes too quickly. I have to go elsewhere. If I am what I think I am, I have to leave this school that I had wanted to go to all my life. I don't belong at Stanford.

I spend a lot of time thinking about where I will go. Then I come up with a crazy plan. I will go to Paris. Gertrude Stein and Alice B. Toklas live there. It must be all right to be a lesbian in Paris. I will go to school at the Sorbonne. I will live among the American expatriates, I will find people like me there. I will find myself.

In April I left Stanford, deeply saddened but resigned to the necessity of it. I applied to the Sorbonne for the fall and went down to Los Angeles to work and wait. My parents had relocated from Tucson to Los Angeles. I told myself that moving in with them was only temporary. I promised myself I would not get caught up in the tangled web of their marriage again.

Yes, my father agreed. If I worked until fall and saved my money, he would match whatever I saved so I could go to Europe. My father rarely kept his promises, but I wanted desperately to believe this time would be different. I made plans accordingly. Of course I couldn't tell anyone why I wanted to go to Paris, but when I was accepted at the Sorbonne that seemed reason enough for everyone.

"Bookkeeper Wanted," the sign in the bookstore window read. I knew nothing about bookkeeping and math was my worst subject, but I loved the idea of working in a bookstore, especially one at the corner of Hollywood and Vine, in those days a glamorous location. The Satyr Bookstore had been a famous hangout for writers like Henry Miller, who was rumored to have actually lived under the staircase in the bookstore a long time ago. What I liked best about working at the Satyr was the chance to sell books, which I did when a clerk was sick or on vacation. I learned the book business there not having a clue that I would spend many years of my life later selling books in other shops, including my own.

Though I was enchanted with bookselling, another job opportunity soon presented itself that I couldn't ignore, particularly one that involved living away from my parents. I had no idea what I was getting into when I agreed to work for the rest of the summer at the Golden State Meat Packing Company.

My father's friend Phil owned the rural meatpacking plant up the coast from Los Angeles in the little town of Santa Maria. Phil needed a bookkeeper for the summer. The job paid well and I would have no expenses, freeing me to save for my European trip. The most intriguing part was that during the week I would stay in Santa Maria.

Phil lived in Beverly Hills with his wife and children. In the early morning darkness every Monday, Phil drove the 150 miles to Santa Maria, where he stayed until Friday, when he returned to his family. The idea was that I would commute with Phil, who in his early forties was an old man to my twenty-year-old mind. Phil dressed like a Beverly Hills cowboy—pressed Levi's, crisp fine-stitched shirt, beautifully hand-tooled boots. He was a handsome man with a full head of sandy blond hair and a tanned, rugged face. He was my father's friend and I felt safe with him.

The big Chrysler Town and Country station wagon bumped over the dirt road and through the gates of the Golden State Meat Packing Company, stopping abruptly in front of a ramshackle white farm house.

"This is where we live," Phil announced cheerfully.

I sat still in the car, my eye drawn to the corrals a few feet away where cattle and hogs milled restlessly, noisily mooing and oinking.

"Does that go on all the time?" I asked.

"All the time," Phil answered.

"How do you sleep?"

"You get used to it."

The stench was like nothing I had ever smelled before, a rich mixture of cow dung, hog excretions, sweat, and something else, the smell of death. I asked what the other buildings were.

"The offices and the kill floor. Want to see it?"

"Not just yet."

The reality of what I'd gotten into began to hit me. I was about to live and work in a slaughterhouse. Somehow it hadn't occurred to me that the Golden State Meat Packing Company was about slaughtering animals. I was immediately sorry, but I took a deep breath and followed Phil into the house. He showed me to my bedroom.

"Where's yours?" I asked.

"Right next to yours," he answered.

I unpacked and cautiously went outside to explore. Across a barren patch of dirt from the house there was something that looked like a loading dock, where a lone figure sat on a chair leaning back against the wall. He was thin and leather-skinned; his broad-brimmed hat had slipped over his eyes.

"Hi," I said. "I'm the new bookkeeper."

The man tipped his hat back and squinted at me through slits of eyes.

"Indian Joe," he mumbled.

I realized that this man was quite drunk. Within a few hours I met the whole crew. Rafe was a giant Swiss-Portuguese, burly and powerful with a soft, gentle voice. Doc, the U.S. Department of Agriculture vet who monitored the killing and butchering, was a short, stocky man with a round, red, angry face. He wore a knee-length white coat with multicolored pens sticking out of his breast pocket. Portuguese Joe was big and fat and bellicose in his blood-stained floor-length apron that he kicked with his boots every time he took a step. Indian Joe was drunk on that first day and every day after that.

I was fascinated by, and a bit scared of, this rough-hewn cast of characters, different from anyone I'd ever come in contact with. I watched everything they did with interest. By contrast they seemed to have no interest in me at all, which was, in its way, a relief.

The day at Golden State began with a predawn breakfast in town with Phil and ended with an evening riding around on dusty country roads so Phil could listen to the baseball game on the car radio. Sometimes we went to a movie in Lompoc or San Luis Obispo. Though I was getting bored with baseball, which I wasn't very interested in to start with, I was okay with our routine. Being in the country was so very different for me; the closest I'd ever come to it was the Stanford "farm." I loved the peacefulness, the way everything seemed to stand still as though waiting for something to happen. Then, one night, something did.

I was just falling asleep when I heard a frantic scratching outside my window. I got up to look, but there was nothing there. I went back to bed, and the scratching started again.

"Phil, do you hear something outside?"

"No, I don't hear anything."

The noise again, louder.

"I sure wish I knew what that is."

"You sound scared. Do you want me to come in there?"

"No. I think I'll just close the window."

The next night the same thing happened—same dialogue, same resolution. It happened night after night. Phil said it was probably just an animal scratching around. One night it got louder and louder as though some creature was trying desperately to break through the wall. I asked Phil if he could hear it.

"No," he said, but again he offered to come to my room to investigate.

"No," I said. "I'll be all right." I didn't want to act like a frightened female, but I also didn't want Phil in my room.

One morning I was playing with the dog that lived on the grounds, throwing a ball that the dog caught in midair. On one throw, he missed and the ball rolled along toward the house. Running after it, I stopped short. There was something sticking to the screen on my window. Examining it more closely, I saw that it was a safety pin hooked to the screen. Tied to the safety pin was a string. I followed the string alongside the house to where it ran into Phil's bedroom window.

With a start I realized what had been happening. Phil would lie in bed and pull on the string to produce the scratching noise that was supposed to frighten me into calling for his help. Once in my bedroom he was better positioned for a seduction that could occur in the context of his rescue mission. I couldn't believe this grown man, my father's friend, was playing such a game with me. After that, no matter how vigorously Phil pulled on his string, I ignored it. One night he almost pulled the screen out of its frame.

"I hear that noise now. Do you want me to come in there?" he'd say.

"No. I'm going to sleep now. Good night." I turned over, smiling.

The string game soon stopped. Phil began going out after our evenings together. He was obviously moving on to the local women since my presence was not going to offer the kind of summer diversion he had been hoping for. I was relieved.

Gradually, I moved closer to the kill floor, first spending time on the loading dock just outside, later standing on tiptoe to peer through the small window in the metal door. I couldn't see much, but the sounds were horrendous—the crack of the rifle, the whirring of machinery, and the whoosh of something liquid that I could only imagine was blood. One day Rafe caught me peeking in the window. He put his hand on my shoulder. "C'mon, I'll take you inside."

I didn't want to go, but Rafe held the door open, beckoning for me to move. I stepped into the half-dark cavern of the kill floor. The smell was overpowering. There was blood everywhere. Rafe leaned down and shouted in my ear, "Watch that chute high up on the wall there."

I heard the crack of a rifle and almost immediately a carcass slid through the opening and bumped awkwardly down the chute. Portuguese Joe grabbed the animal's leg and quickly attached it to a chain that hoisted it upside down to glide along a track until it rested over a large, round, metal container. With one deft movement, Joe slit the animal's throat and held the body steady as the blood poured into the bleeding tank. The process was swift and efficient.

Rafe explained the next steps, then pushed me toward the giant walk-in freezer at one end of the room. He opened the door to a mist-shrouded sepulcher where headless carcasses hung. This was the end of the line, the last stop before USDA inspection and the journey to market and table. I found myself thinking that I would never eat meat again.

Rafe turned me back to the kill floor and was guiding me toward a piece of equipment that consisted of rows of huge, whirling roller brushes. Big, black, hairy hog carcasses were being fed into one end of the dehairing machine, emerging from the other end smooth, pink, and glistening. It happened so fast it was fascinating.

The kill-floor workers nonchalantly went about their business, their booted feet sloshing through puddles of blood, the din of the dehairing machine in their ears as they hoisted, sliced, and hacked away, shouting to one another, joking and laughing. I trust that more modern meatpacking plants are operated in a much less blood-and-guts atmosphere than this rural slaughterhouse was in the 1940s.

To that point, death was something I'd had no reason to think about, but in that setting I began to think about how much it is a part of life. We kill these creatures so that we can go on living. I thought about becoming a vegetarian, but I knew that wouldn't put an end to the killing, nothing would. This cycle was a contract with nature: certain creatures kill others in order to survive. It was necessary for balance . . . wasn't it?

I was proud of myself for going onto the kill floor and not fleeing in horror. I proved myself, though for what I'm not sure. After my first visit, I was able to return to the kill floor occasionally when I had to talk to someone there or just to convince myself that I could. But when the summer was over, I was quite ready to move on to the rest of my life.

Children often have fantasies about their parents, seeing them as the people they want them to be rather than the people they are. Adult children do it, too. I had a fantasy father—caring, honest, and dependable—but my father was none of those things. When the time came for him to keep his promise to match what I had earned so I could travel to Europe, he reneged. It was as though he'd never made the commitment. The parallel reality he operated in did not include sensitivity to the feelings and needs of the people around him.

I was furious at yet another betrayal, another message to me that what I wanted didn't matter to either of my parents. I felt a deep sadness as I realized that it was really time for me to cut the cord, to no longer look to these people for support of any kind. I needed to get away from my egocentric parents if I were ever to learn to see myself as a worthwhile individual, deserving enough to matter to anyone. Paris was out. I couldn't afford it. I substituted Greenwich Village and set out for the East Coast. I was scared but determined to make it on my own.

3

I had dated Monroe in high school. His parents lived in Tucson, but he went to military school in another state, which gave him a certain cachet. We spent time together on holidays and during the summer. Now his family had moved back to New York, so Monroe was the person I looked to for help as I made my lonely pilgrimage eastward. He found me a room in Greenwich Village in a shabby hotel, but the price seemed right.

On the night of my arrival, Monroe appeared, loaded down with maps, subway schedules, and pamphlets describing what to see in New York. He spread everything out on the bed and began to explain the city from the Bowery to the Bronx. By the time he left, at least I knew what I needed to know to navigate Manhattan.

Excited, I went to bed and was just falling asleep when the first crash resounded in the next room. A man's voice shouted obscenities, a woman screamed, a door slammed and someone sobbed loudly. I was terrified. Was someone being murdered? I called the desk and got a rather bored clerk, who said not to worry, no one was being murdered, and the noise would stop soon. It did, for that night, but the performance was repeated night after night. When it started I just closed my eyes and waited. It never occurred to me to ask to have my room changed. I just accepted it as part of the sound and fury of New York City.

One of the greatest challenges of my initial adjustment to Manhattan was the subway. Thunder in a cave, the trains roared into the station, stopping so briefly I wondered how I would ever be able to jump on without getting crushed as the doors slammed shut. I stood poised to dash when the next train stopped and the doors opened to disgorge a mob of people. I pushed past them just as the doors slammed and the train hurtled into the darkness.

Monroe had told me to be ever alert for my stop on the subway or I would be riding a long time. I watched wide-eyed as the signs whizzed by. When we got close to the Forties, I positioned myself by the door, ready to push my way out. Forty-second Street. The car lurched to a stop. I was barely on the platform when the train roared away. My head was reeling. Upstairs, the daylight was a very welcome sight.

The streets of New York are a miracle of cacophony—horns honking, taxi drivers cursing, the metal lifts of trucks crashing down, delivery people screaming indecipherable reprimands into the air. The midtown sidewalks were an endless stream of walkers flowing in both directions. I stepped into the stream and was immediately carried forward. When I lost my concentration and drifted into the oncoming foot traffic, I was rudely jostled back into my own lane. It took several weeks of this sport for me to play the game without feeling that I was at risk for being run over. Eventually I was able to glide along with the crowd like a pro.

One day I was walking along Forty-seventh Street when I came upon the Gotham Book Mart. I didn't know that it was one of the most famous book stores in all the world. I stepped inside and was startled to see such a profusion of books—jam-packed shelves floor to ceiling, books piled on tables and stacked on carts in the aisles, books and books everywhere. What a wonderful place to work this would be. I asked for the owner and was approached by a diminutive woman with graying hair, pale skin, blue eyes, and a stern demeanor.

"What is it?" she asked in a testy voice.

I said I was applying for a job, that I'd had experience selling books at the Satyr Bookstore in Hollywood. She motioned me to one of the two little wooden stools in front of the cash register. We sat.

"What kind of books did you sell?"

I did a quick survey of the shelves near me. "All kinds, but mostly avant-garde, like this."

"You're awfully young. Where is your family?"

"In Los Angeles. I just got here."

"Where are you living?"

"The University Place Hotel."

She shuddered. "Too seedy and too expensive. Get an apartment."

"I will if you give me this job."

Frances Steloff lowered her head and looked up at me through bushy eyebrows. After a long minute, she spoke. "When can you start?"

"Tomorrow."

"Be here promptly at eight. I don't like tardiness. You're on trial for one month, $25 a week. Wear sensible shoes." And with that Frances Steloff got up and walked away. I couldn't believe I had pulled it off so easily. I was ecstatic.

I reported for work the next morning eager to learn the stock I would be selling. Wrong. I wasn't going to *sell* books; I was going to *carry* them. I carried books up from the basement and down to the basement, all day long, up the stairs and down the stairs. I worked under the supervision of Horace, a strapping young black man. He would often follow me up and down the stairs as I staggered under the weight of huge stacks of books. I weighed in at about ninety pounds then, all five feet of me. Horace, a six-footer, never offered to carry a single book. I went home every night exhausted and irritated but determined to stick it out.

One of the most intriguing things about the Gotham Book Mart was the basement where row upon row of pristine first editions of James Joyce, Ernest Hemingway, Gertrude Stein, T. S. Eliot, Henry Miller, and Thomas Wolfe were stashed. For years Frances Steloff had been buying large quantities of first editions of authors she predicted would be successful. She stored the books until the authors became literary stars, after which she sold the mint first editions at a premium price. She seemed to have an unerring eye for those writers who would become winners. Gore Vidal said of her, "She had an instinct about who was going to be duly noted in time, that was her specific genius."

The other great source of excitement at the GBM was the parade of literary and theatrical celebrities who patronized the store. In the first month I worked there I saw W. H. Auden, Marianne Moore, Elizabeth Bishop, Gore Vidal, and Eugene O'Neill. Of course Miss Steloff waited on them herself, but by then I was actually selling books. I had passed my probationary period and graduated to clerking for the several hours of the day I was not hauling books up and down the stairs.

Although I was thrilled about selling books I was also troubled by the oppressive way Miss Steloff hovered over each sale. She wore the only key to the cash register on a short chain around her neck, like a skate key. When a sale was made by any clerk, she would materialize to open the register, bending over nearly double. She would take the money, make the change, then hand it to the clerk to pass to the customer.

It was known that she owned the GBM building, and it was rumored that she was landlord to even more of the Forty-seventh Street block. Yet, she lived alone in an apartment above the store. Seated on one of the two wooden stools in front of the cash register, she would eat her lunch, birdlike, from a brown paper bag. Miss Steloff was frugal to a fault, a strange and fascinating character who opened up the world of bookselling to me even as I was learning from her a distinct lesson on how not to live as a person. It is likely that she had sources of great enjoyment in her days and nights that I knew nothing about, but what I mainly saw in her was a great sense of weariness.

Believing that my position at GBM was established, I went hunting for an apartment in Greenwich Village. I found a place that seemed like heaven to me, a first-floor front in a converted brownstone on Twelfth Street. It had floor-to-ceiling windows; a large, ornate chandelier; and a working fireplace framed in marble. There was a tiny kitchen, a bed, a couch, a table, and four chairs. That was it, all I needed.

I couldn't believe the rent was only $50 a month, utilities included. Fabulous! My salary was $100 a month. I could afford that. Needless to say, I didn't know that one shouldn't spend fifty percent of one's total income on housing. It wasn't until I was out on the street that I realized I'd seen no bathroom. There had to be a bathroom. There was—down the hall, shared with three other apartments. No matter, I had a chandelier and a working fireplace. I moved in the next day and was deliriously happy, living in New York and working at the Gotham Book Mart. What more could a person want?

"Dummkopf!" the book came flying through the air and crashed into the side of my head. "Look behind! Look behind!"

I was stunned. I'd not been able to find the book a customer was asking for. I'd forgotten there were books *behind* books. I pulled out the first row and did indeed find what he wanted. Smarting from the blow to my head and to my pride, I brought the book to Miss Steloff and hurried away, feeling tears coming. When the customer was gone I told Miss Steloff I could not tolerate having books thrown at my head. She said that was fine and maybe I'd like to work someplace else. She opened the cash register and handed me a week's pay. Once out the door my tears came in a torrent.

I felt like a failure. What should I have done? Was I really that stupid? Should I have quit? I had tried so hard to be a willing student, an enthusiastic apprentice. Why had she treated me that way? It didn't occur to me at the time that I had not failed, that I had simply been the victim of an eccentric woman's temper tantrum. It did help, some years later, to hear that another

GOTHAM BOOK MART

DEAR MISS BERZON: Frances Steloff

YOUR LETTER CAME IN THE MIDST OF CHRISTMAS RUSH AND THEN
CAME INVENTORY SO THIS HAS BEEN MY FIRST OPPORTUNITY TO
WRITE YOU. I HAVE SINCE HEARD HOW ATTRACTIVE YOUR SHOP
IS AND THE GBM FLAVOR THAT PERMEATES IT. WE HAVE A
GREAT MANY THINGS IN SMALL QUANTITIES THAT WE COULD SHARE
WITH YOU BUT THERE IS A PROBLEM OF FINANCE.

WE HAVE COOPERATED MORE THAN ONCE WITH PEOPLE ON THE COAST
AND HAVE LOST SOMETIMES QUITE HEAVILY. THE LARRY EDMUND'S
BOOKSHOP TO WHOM WE SENT A VERY CHOICE ORDER REMAINS UNPAID
AND SINCE THEY HAVE CHANGED HANDS THERE IS LITTLE HOPE
THAT WE SHALL GET PAID. A FREE LANCE BOOKSELLER BY NAME
LILLIAN BLOOD OWES US SEVERAL HUNDRED DOLLARS. WE HOLD
NOTES BUT THAT'S ALL THE GOOD IT HAS DONE US. OTHERS WE
COULD MENTION BUT THE POINT IS WE ARE NOT WILLING TO
TAKE ANY MORE CHANCES. IF YOU LIKE WE COULD SEND YOU A
SAMPLE ORDER OF ONE EACH OF A DOZEN ITEMS WHICH WOULD NOT
RUN INTO VERY MUCH AND YOU COULD THEN JUDGE WHETHER WE CAN
DEAL TOGETHER.

A FEW LISTS SELECTED HURRIEDLY AT RANDOM AND ARE STOCK
WITH WHICH YOU ARE MORE OR LESS FAMILIAR MIGHT BE SUFFICIENT
LEADS. MEANWHILE THE BEST OF GOOD LUCK. WE HAVE OFTEN
BEEN URGED TO START A BRANCH AND THEY ALL SEEM TO THINK
THERE IS ROOM FOR A GBM JR. SO YOU CAN FILL THE NEED.

MISS KIEL SAW YOUR LETTER AND REMEMBERS YOU VERY WELL
AND SENDS GOOD WISHES.

WITH ALL GOOD WISHES.

JANUARY 20, 1951.

BERZON BOOKS
1645 N. LAS PALMAS
HOLLYWOOD 28, CALIF.

SINCERELY,
Frances Steloff per SL
GOTHAM BOOK MART

41 WEST 47th STREET · NEW YORK · PLAZA 7-0367,8 · CABLE 'GOTHMART'

A letter from Frances Steloff complimenting my bookstore. I doubt that Frances
remembered how I precipitously left her employ at Gotham Book Mart
after she threw a book at my head when I couldn't find the volume
a customer was asking for.

"dummkopf" had been fired from the GBM under exactly the same conditions after he could not find what a customer asked for and a book had been thrown at his head. His name was Tennessee Williams.

Surprisingly, that was not my last contact with Frances Steloff. In years to come I visited the store several times, and she always claimed she remembered me, though I doubt that was true. I only felt truly redeemed when some years later Miss Steloff wrote me a letter congratulating me on opening my own bookstore in Hollywood. She said she had heard the store was attractive, that it had a GBM flavor, and that it could be the Gotham Book Mart Junior of the West Coast. It was a warm, gracious letter, and I was sure she didn't realize she was writing to one of the dummkopfs she'd thrown a book at and fired. The last time I saw Frances Steloff she was ninety-eight, still working in the store, though she had given up her skate key, and still living upstairs. When she died, at 101, the *Los Angeles Times* described her in a long obituary as "America's most venerated bookseller."

In the autumn of 1948 I sat in my darkened apartment, panicked that I had no job and no income and the rent was due in a week. I'd looked for a job, but no luck. I was eating in the Automat or skipping meals, trying to hang on to what was left of my dwindling savings. Maybe this was a fool's mission I was on, alone in a tough city, no family, one friend. I probably had no business being in New York at all. Maybe I wasn't ready to take care of myself. I cried in despair, feeling hopeless.

When the phone rang, I jumped. The voice on the other end said, "Hi. This is Susan. I'm here."

"Here? Where?"

"Right here in New York. I'm finished at Stanford and I'm home."

"But Susan, you're only a junior. How could you be finished?"

"I accelerated, took a lot of honors courses. I think they wanted to get rid of me. They don't like pushy New Yorkers at Stanford."

Susan certainly was pushy, something I'd liked about her when we became friends, pushy and smart.

"Okay, I'm here now, done with school. How are you?"

I took a deep breath. "I'm great. I have a terrific job and a swell apartment. I'm having a wonderful time."

"Super. Where do you live? I'm coming over."

"Uh, I have plans for tonight."

"Fine. I'll come for half an hour. What's the address?"

I stammered out the address and she hung up. Time to pull myself together. Turn on the lights. Wear something upbeat. Put on a happy face. Figure out what to talk about. Make coffee. Play music. And then Susan was knocking on the door.

Ten minutes into Susan's questions about my life she had guessed the truth. She wanted to know the exact state of my finances, and I told her everything.

"I've got the answer," Susan said with her usual self-assurance. "I have a friend, Judith, known her since grammar school, just broke up with her boyfriend and needs a place to live. She's an actress, nice person, has money for rent, you'll like her. I'll call right now."

Within the hour Judith was there. She was startlingly beautiful with a honey-soft voice and a pleasant, graceful manner. I told her my situation and she offered to move in and pay the rent until I was working again. I couldn't believe it. I was instantly beholden, grateful, and to my dismay, smitten. She opened the door to the outside hall and there was her luggage, which she had brought with her. Was it optimism, desperation, or just plain New York chutzpah? It didn't matter. She moved in and I was thrilled.

Judith was as smart as she was beautiful, and over the next few weeks we spoke of many things. I loved being with her. There was, however, one rather distracting problem. We had only one bed and Judith slept in the nude. I tried not to look at her. I slept on the very edge of my side, almost falling out of bed night after night. I was acutely aware of her presence mere inches away. It did not make for peaceful sleeping.

One night I went out to a party where I had more than my share of wine. I began to think about Judith. I couldn't get her out of my mind. Whatever defenses I'd been able to muster in denying my attraction to her were suddenly gone. I called the apartment and said that I had something to tell her and I was coming right home. No time for the subway, I hailed a cab. Never mind that I was using several of my last dollars.

The taxi seemed to take forever. When we arrived at my building, I shoved money at the driver and jumped out. As the taxi sped away I realized I'd left my purse in the cab. What was happening to me? Had I lost my mind?

Judith was sitting up in bed, smiling pleasantly, curious about what I was going to tell her. I was very nervous. I sat down on the bed and took Judith's hand. With great trepidation, I leaned over and kissed her on the mouth. She did not kiss me back.

"Judith, I think I'm in love with you," I blurted out.

She withdrew her hand.

"Well," she said, "I'm very flattered, but you know I don't swing that way. I hope I haven't done anything to cause you to think I do. If I have, I apologize."

She got off the bed and crossed the room. I watched her light a cigarette.

"I think you are very nice," she was saying, "and I really like you as a friend. Maybe it would be best if I moved."

"Moved?"

"I think it would be best."

In half an hour she was packed. It was obviously something she was accustomed to doing in a hurry. She carried her bags into the hall and came back in. "I'm really sorry," she said. Leaning over, she kissed me gently on the cheek. Then she was gone.

I felt as though I had just made the biggest mistake of my life, inviting rejection and ridicule. But she had not ridiculed me. She had actually been very gentle in her rejection. Yet even that made me feel pitiable. I hated what had happened. I hated myself.

There is something unnerving about putting the key in the door of one's apartment and finding that it doesn't turn. I looked around to make sure I was in the right building. It never occurred to me that the locks had been changed. I went looking for the super. Cracking his door a few inches, he peered out at me. I told him there was a problem with my apartment door.

"No problem with your door. Problem's with your rent. It hasn't been paid, two weeks over due. Locks changed."

I was horrified. All of my things were in the apartment. Where would I sleep? I pleaded with him. "Please. Please. I'll get the money in a few days. I promise. Oh please." I think it was the tears that got to him.

"Awright. I shouldn't, but you get that money to me right away. Here's the key. Now don't bother me no more tonight."

The next day I went out determined to get a job, and I did. Burt Franklin, Inc., was a mail-order book business operating out of an enormous loft on Wall Street. Cataloging books was tedious, and eating lunch at the crowded stand-up counters was perilous, considering my face was at the same level as everyone else's flying elbows, but the people I worked with were pleasant and I sometimes went out with them for drinks after work.

One night we went to a bar we hadn't been to before. Behind the bar was something unusual: a wooden box was attached to the wall. It had a screen on which a movie was being shown. I looked around for the projector, but there was none. I asked the bartender where the projector was.

"There is no projector. I don't know how they do it, but it's called 'television.'"

We all sat transfixed, watching the murky images move across the screen. Who would have thought that this little movie-in-a-box would someday be the most powerful conduit in history for shaping the attitudes and habits of an entire planet?

If Susan knew anything about what had happened with Judith she never mentioned it. Instead, she did what she had done at Stanford, lobby me to lose my precious virginity. Unlike most young women in the 1940s, Susan had no inhibitions when it came to sex. She loved sleeping with men, and she thought I should be doing the same. Her litany would start: "You are ridiculous. What are you saving it for? Sex is fun. You're too old to be a virgin!"

My resistance to Susan's campaign was at a low ebb. I felt embarrassed about Judith and confused about what I was doing with my life. Maybe I should not be exploring my attraction to women. I didn't seem to be very good at it. So far I'd just made a damn fool of myself. Susan's timing was excellent. Just as I was reconsidering my sexual options, she produced the "perfect" candidate with whom to lose my virginity.

Jay was a Yale law student. His parents were friends of Susan's parents. He was single, and Susan seemed to know that he was also horny. At dinner Jay droned on about himself and his family. His invitation to his parents' place was inevitable, since he had already established that they were out of town. At the apartment, we were into our second glass of champagne when, without warning, he pulled me off the couch and led me down the hallway to a bedroom. I was startled at the suddenness of it.

In the bedroom he pushed me down on the bed and began unbuttoning my blouse. All I could think was, "Okay, this is what I'm supposed to be doing." Jay was out of his clothes and on top of me, kissing my throat, my breasts, my mouth—no words spoken. I lay there passively, disconnected, watching as though it were happening to someone else. I was aware, however, that I was not ready for this. Then Jay began to penetrate, not looking at me. I thought, "He doesn't even know I'm here. I'm just a body to him; this has nothing to do with me." Suddenly, I seemed to wake up.

"Wait. Stop. This is my first time. Please stop."

Jay stopped. He scrutinized my face. "C'mon, forget that stuff. This isn't your first time. You were too easy." And he resumed his performance.

I continued to murmur in a small voice, "Please, no, stop." I tried not to think about what was happening to me, the pain, the anger, the helplessness. It felt like such an alien experience, an invasion against which I had no defense.

It was quickly over. Jay rolled off of me, and I stared at the ceiling. After a minute I said, "I'd like some more champagne." Jay didn't answer. I turned to look at him; he was sound asleep. The term "date rape" didn't exist then nor did the concept. Jay's behavior was not at all unusual for what young males in that era were taught about sex: You should want it. You should get it. Satisfy yourself. Don't take no for an answer. Women like to have sex forced upon them. No means yes.

Jay was right. I was too easy. I was using him as he was using me. It was Susan I should have a beef with. No, I was the one who created this mess, seeking to be "normal," having no idea what that really meant for me or for anybody else.

"Oh, just forget it," Susan said. "You got it over with and that's what's important. Now, I've got a wonderful guy for you to meet, nothing like Jay, a real mensch. I'm arranging a date."

Si was a reporter on a small suburban newspaper. Boyish and impish looking, he was easy to like and fun to be with. With Si there was no agenda as there had been with Jay. We got to know each other slowly, talking about books, enjoying our mutual interests. On our third date, Si took me to a charming, below-street-level restaurant in the Village called the Salle de Champagne. I'd passed it many times, peering down through the window at the people dining in the warm glow of candlelight.

We had a lovely dinner and were feeling quite mellow as we climbed the stairs to the sidewalk where we stopped in our tracks. The sky was bright red and the air was thick with smoke. Coughing and straining to see through the haze, we could make out flames shooting into the sky about a block away. Si shouted, "C'mon, let's go!" and we ran in the direction of the fire. We were stopped at the corner by a police officer.

"You can't go any further."

Si flashed his press card, and we were passed immediately through the police barrier. The inferno raged in front of us, a block-long building totally engulfed in flames. Fire trucks lined the street and firemen were running in all directions, hauling their hoses, shouting above the roar of the fire. Waves of heat rolled toward us as we stood facing the burning building. The sound of the fire was like the cracking of thunder. Si said something that I didn't hear to a fireman who yelled back, "It's a hat factory. We don't think anyone is in there, but we're not sure."

At that moment a great whoosh of water bounced off the building and splashed across the narrow street, soaking us. Si held tightly to my hand. "Are you okay?" he shouted.

"Yes, yes, I'm fine."

I was wet all over, my eyes burned, my heart was pounding, and I couldn't breathe, but I was strangely exhilarated. I felt drawn by the fire, pulled into its center. I was disappointed when, after half an hour, the flames began to subside. Si was pulling at me. I couldn't hear what he was saying, but his lips formed the words, "Let's go." I let him lead me away from the building.

As we walked toward my apartment, I had a feeling of sadness. I didn't want this adventure to end. I could still hear the fire crackling in my ears. I had liked feeling the danger and the heat. I wanted the excitement to continue, but I didn't tell Si what I was feeling. I was afraid he would think I was crazy.

One night, Si said he had to deliver something to his parents' apartment and would I mind if we did it before going to dinner. Taking a taxi rather than our usual subway train, I was surprised when we turned into Park Avenue and stopped in front of a canopied entrance. A uniformed doorman opened the door of the cab, tipped his hat, and said, "Good evening, Mr. Newhouse."

In the apartment, Si explained that his parents were in Europe and he was sorry I couldn't meet them, then he disappeared. I looked around at the tasteful elegance of the room I was in, the softly lit art, the beautiful colors and textures, the muted richness. I got it. Si Newhouse was not just a young reporter on a suburban newspaper.

That night, I asked Si what his father did. "He's in the communications business," was all he would say. After that, I felt less comfortable with Si, as though there was something important I didn't know, privileged information, or was it information about privilege? He chose not to talk about his father's substantial wealth or the potential he had to become as powerful as his father. Perhaps he was just shaping his own identity at the time, but somehow I got the feeling that it would always be difficult to really get into Si. He would control the access, and I would be allowed to move only where he wanted me to. Eventually, we drifted apart, both of us in periods of exploring the options of our lives.

1962. I picked up an issue of *Time* and there on the cover was S. I. Newhouse, Sr., Si's father, whose "communications business" was a jaw-dropping media empire that included newspapers, magazines, television stations, and publishing companies. Inside I saw a picture of the family— mother Mitzi, father Sam, married brother Donald, and unmarried Si. I was very interested in the unmarried part.

What I remembered about Si in 1962, thirteen years after the fact, was that we had some good times together. Maybe I should review this relationship. Perhaps I missed something. I phoned New York and found it surprisingly easy to reach Si, who remembered me and invited me to call him when I am in town. A week later, I was in New York, opening the door of my hotel room to Si Newhouse, no longer the impish twenty-year-old, but a rather serious-looking fellow in a gray three-piece suit. I was glad to see him, promising myself not to be intimidated by anything I heard from him. That turned out to be not so easy.

I asked Si what's new, probably a silly question to ask after thirteen years. He answered quickly that the most exciting thing happening was that his father had just bought his mother a thirty-fifth wedding-anniversary gift, the Condé Nast publications. I was speechless, but I managed to say, "How nice."

I saw that this was not going to be an easy evening. We dined at 21, not downstairs with the crowd but upstairs in a private room, deadly quiet, ours the only table, served by a swarm of waiters. From the bowing and scraping that went on it was obvious that Si was a well-known and valued patron. He ordered the dinner in advance, so there were no decisions to be made.

At dinner Si talked about his mother, Mitzi, who wore a size three, and the likelihood that size three would become the standard for fashion models in the future. Because the family then owned *Vogue, Mademoiselle, Glamour,* and *Vanity Fair,* I assumed he knew what he was talking about.

I searched Si's face for any signs of the Si I knew, the venturesome young man who courted danger by pulling me into a raging inferno just for the thrill of being there. I didn't see that young man, but I was heartened when he suggested that we go someplace else after dinner. My mind ran to the Peppermint Lounge, home of the Twist, which I'd just learned to do, or maybe a Greenwich Village club, where a sensational new young singer named Bob Dylan was appearing.

Si said, "I was thinking of Rizzoli's."

"Rizzoli's? Fine." After all, I didn't know the name of every bar in New York.

I was soon clued in as we entered Rizzoli's Bookstore. There was a respectful hush as browsers moved silently among the shelves. I love books, but in 1962 this was not my idea of a night on the town in New York City. It was clear that Si and I were worlds apart, strangers. Whatever connected us once was only a fond memory.

I have followed Si's career with interest, given that his spectacular success is frequently reported in the press. *Forbes Magazine* once described Si and his brother as the fifth richest men in America. Together they added Random House, Alfred Knopf, Crown, the *New Yorker,* and numerous other choice properties to the media empire they inherited from their father.

But I remember with affection that boyish young reporter, the one who didn't want to talk about who his father was or what he did, the one who didn't seem to know who he was yet or what he was going to become.

It wasn't like you could look in the phone book under "L" to find lesbians in 1949. I didn't know where to start. I probably didn't even want to start, but ultimately this is why I'd come to New York. I had to do something. There was a bar on MacDougal Street called Terry's. I'd passed it a few times and seen some rather masculine-looking women emerging. Maybe . . .

I stood in front of Terry's Bar and peered in the window. The scene inside was wall-to-wall women: young, old, standing, sitting, drinking, smoking, talking. In the flickering light of the table candles I could see that some of the women were dressed like men. I was shivering. The night was cold. Was it the chill outside or the panic I felt inside watching this scene? I pressed my nose against the glass to see better. I felt like a child watching a room full of grown-ups, set apart, drawn to something forbidden. I watched with fascination and dread, wanting to be inside but too frightened to even know how I could get there.

Peering through that window I suddenly felt self-conscious. What if someone saw me? What if someone thought I was just staring at the weirdos inside? What if someone inside saw me and thought I was a crazy person who might do them harm? What was I doing? Why was I there? What was wrong with me? Too confused to make sense of myself, I backed away and hurried down the street.

In the ensuing weeks, thoughts of Terry's Bar played in my mind. I wanted to go back, but for what? Did I belong there? I couldn't picture myself inside that room. It wasn't just a bar to me; it felt more like a black hole into which I could be lost forever. I was terrified of it, but I couldn't get it out of my mind.

What I did instead was immerse myself in a social life that was familiar and felt safe, with men. Two of my most important friends were Adam Margoshus and Seymour Hacker, with whom I had one of the more memorable encounters of my New York life. Adam owned a small bookstore in the Village, and Seymour was the proprietor of a respected art gallery on Fifty-seventh Street. Seymour was diminutive, but he had the commanding presence of a person accustomed to having his authority taken seriously. Adam looked like a menacing giant, shaggy, uncombed, often unshaven, in a dyed-black army-issue great coat. He was an imposing figure, but he was sweet, gentle, and one of the smartest people I have ever met.

New Years Eve, 1949. Adam, Seymour, and I go together to a huge blow-out of a party in an artist's loft in the Village, plenty of beer, cheap wine, very loud music, and hordes of people. It is late, already into the new year, and the noise level in the room is deafening, but I am enjoying the shouting match that passes for a conversation I am having with a very Ivy League–looking young man whose name I never catch.

Seymour pushes his way through the crowd to me and shouts in my ear, "I'm ready to leave this place. I'm invited to another party. Wanna go?" I nod affirmatively.

"Can I bring him?" I ask, pointing to Ivy League.

"Sure, why not?" Seymour shouts. "I'll go and get Adam and we'll meet at the front door."

I take Ivy League's hand and he follows me, apparently happy to be tagging along, though he does look rather startled when he sees Adam. We make our way to the subway, and on the ride uptown I ask Seymour where we are going.

"Tallulah Bankhead's," he says.

We all stare at him.

"I met her the other night and she invited me to this party," Seymour says, answering a question that hadn't been asked. I'm thrilled. I'd just seen Tallulah in *Private Lives* a few nights before, and I adored her.

We bypass the unattended reception desk of the Hotel Elysee. That should have been a clue that the night was giving way to morning, but we were too into our adventure to think about what time it was. Seymour seems to know exactly where he is going. Our little band pauses at Miss Bankhead's door, adjusting clothes, smoothing hair, straightening glasses. Seymour knocks. No answer. He knocks again, louder. We can hear some hurried conversation inside, then silence. Seymour knocks again. Suddenly the door is thrown wide open and framed against the light is a tall, gorgeous young man, stark naked, from whom emanates the unmistakable *odeur* of sex. I recognize him immediately as the actor I saw in *Private Lives* with Miss Bankhead.

"What is it?" he demands crossly.

Seymour pulls himself up to his full five feet five inches and speaks in his most authoritative voice. "I have been invited to a party here by Miss Bankhead. Is she available?"

The young man slams the door in our faces. Seymour is furious, sputtering with anger. "How dare he!" And with that, he pounds on the door with his fist. Again, the door is thrown open.

"Go away or I'll call the police!" the actor says.

Suddenly we all become aware of a sound building somewhere in the deeper reaches of the suite. It is a kind of moaning that grows louder as its source draws nearer. And then, like a locomotive rounding the curve at top speed, the moaning turns into a guttural growl, and she is upon us—Tallulah Bankhead, dressing gown flying, eyes blazing. She pushes the actor out of the way and snarls, "What's going on here?"

We are all speechless.

"Well," she demands, "what do you want?"

Seymour clears his throat. "How do you do, Miss Bankhead. We met the other evening and you invited me to a party here tonight."

"Do you know what time it is?" she roars.

At this point Adam becomes impatient. As he moves toward Tallulah, she takes a step backward.

"Well," Adam asks, "is there a party going on here or isn't there?"

Miss Bankhead studies Adam for a long moment. Then, tossing her head back in the manner of a woman accustomed to having her every gesture attended to, she announces, "There's a party going on here, honey, but you're not going to join it!" And with that, she slams the door with all her might.

We stand there, stunned. Seymour begins sputtering again. Ivy League says, "Just what time is it anyway?" It was only then that we realize it is 5 A.M.

"Let's get some breakfast," Adam says, and he shuffles toward the elevator. Outside, we walk until we find an all-night diner. We silently seat ourselves around a table. No one speaks. Then, almost imperceptibly, a small ripple of laughter escapes from Seymour. Ivy League begins to giggle, too. I look at Adam and we both burst out laughing. Suddenly, we are all laughing, rolling around in our chairs, holding our sides. Seymour raises his water glass and proposes a toast: "Here's to Tallulah, long may she rave!" And we are off again into gales of laughter that subside only with the arrival of the first breakfast of 1950.

4

The first week of 1950 blew in with a bone-chilling blizzard that turned Manhattan into an ordeal of snow and ice. I had never been so cold. The ribs of the tiny electric heater in my apartment glowed red, valiantly trying to warm the high-ceilinged room. I wrapped myself in layers of sweaters and spent my time at home huddled in bed, longing for California, fearing that I would freeze to death and not be found until the spring thaw.

I loved my grand first-floor front, but the impracticality of having no heat was getting to me. I decided it was time to seek warmth. The "For Rent" ads in the local newspaper, the *Villager,* were all for unfurnished apartments. Then my eye fell on "Roommate Wanted: Want quiet, intelligent girl to share my Village apartment." I'd never had a roommate (excluding Judith's brief stay), but why not?

She said, "Come right over."

It was a fifth-floor walk-up right in the middle of Eighth, the busiest, noisiest street in the Village: movie theater right across, nightclub downstairs, restaurants and shops all around. I climbed the five flights, the noise of the street fading as I neared the top. I wasn't ready for the person who answered the door.

Marilyn was quite beautiful, a slim blonde with translucent green eyes in a chiseled face. She invited me in to a room that was almost in darkness. As I felt my way inside I saw that the walls and ceiling were painted black. The carpet was also black. Tiny shafts of light filtered through four dormer windows high up on the wall. Twin black-shaded coolie lamps provided the other illumination, two small pools of light on the table underneath them.

As my eyes adjusted I saw one big room, two studio couches at right angles with a table between, a small kitchen area, and a door I assumed led to a bathroom. What felt most important about this mysterious black interior was its toasty warmth. Marilyn sat on one of the studio couches and patted the other for me to sit down.

"Do you work?" she asked.

"Yes, I work for a direct-mail bookseller in Wall Street."

"Where are you from?"

"Los Angeles."

"Well, me too. How long have you been here?"

"About eight months."

"Planning to stay?"

"For the foreseeable future."

"The rent is $50 a month."

"How much would my share be?"

"Fifty dollars."

"All of it?"

"Of course. I furnished the apartment, in addition to which I am dead broke. I haven't worked for three months."

"What kind of work do you do?"

"I'm a fashion model."

Was it my imagination or was she leaning into the lamplight as though posing? She looked like a model: long torso, long legs, perfectly defined face. I looked around the room, a pretty small space for two people, but the thought of living with someone as glamorous as Marilyn was intriguing.

"Okay, I'll take it. When shall I move in?"

"How about tomorrow?"

"Tomorrow is fine," I said quickly, not giving a thought to how I was going to handle getting out of my present apartment or moving my things.

The next day I hauled suitcases and boxes out to a cab while the driver sat staring straight ahead. On Eighth Street, he again sat motionless behind the wheel while I staggered under my burden. I eliminated the tip and turned away, not quite catching the driver's muttered curse as he screeched from the curb.

I stood on the sidewalk craning my neck to locate the fifth-floor dormers. I was too shy and too embarrassed to ask Marilyn for help, so I made three trips to drag my belongings up the five flights. When she opened the door, Marilyn looked startled.

"How in the world did you get all this stuff up here?"

"Oh, the cab driver helped me."

Marilyn laughed, "Sure he did." She'd obviously lived in New York too long to believe that. When I was unpacked, Marilyn suggested we get some dinner downstairs. I was delighted with that and with her invitation to go out for a drink with some friends who were coming over after dinner.

They arrived in a group: three women and a man, no, not a man, a very tall woman in men's clothes. Marilyn caught me staring.

"Rusty, where is your lipstick?" she asked nervously. The tall woman looked puzzled.

"My what?"

"Lipstick, you know." Marilyn made putting on lipstick motions.

"Oh, yeah, lipstick. I guess I ate it all off at dinner." Rusty grinned foolishly.

It hit me—these women were all lesbians! Marilyn was going to try to conceal that from her straight little roommate. What should I do, go along, play dumb? I couldn't tell them the truth about myself because I didn't even know the truth. What a bizarre turn of events! I answered an ad looking for warmth and I found lesbians!

I walked along silently with the group, glad for the driving snow that made conversation impossible. When we turned into MacDougal Street I knew my fate was sealed. We were headed for Terry's Bar! I had a strange feeling of being out of my body as we approached the door, that formidable barrier I thought I could never get through. Rusty was holding the door for me. Trying to look nonchalant, I took the few steps into the bar, feeling like I was entering a whole new era of my life.

Inside, I followed the group through the haze of smoke to a table. As we sat, Marilyn spoke: "My, look at all these women. It must be ladies' night."

She got looks from her friends but no one said a word. I couldn't believe she was going to do this. Why had she invited me to go out with her friends so quickly? I must have seemed awfully stupid to her. I said nothing.

Soon other women came to our table. Everyone seemed to know everyone else. Marilyn introduced me as her new roommate, pointedly emphasizing that I had answered her ad in the newspaper for someone to share her apartment. People were polite to me but quickly moved on to talk to the others. They all had a lot to say to one another, mostly gossip about who was going with whom, who had broken up, and what terrible things had happened to them at work or with their families. I sat quietly listening, fascinated by what I was hearing but at the same time horrified by their war stories. They spoke of painful experiences, yet without emotion, as though it was all so routine it wasn't worth expending feelings on.

As the alcohol took its toll, another aspect of their history came out— they were all ex-lovers of one another, and remnants of unfinished business among them crept into the conversation. It was almost as though they were speaking in code, as families do, fragments of sentences conveying volumes of emotion. Entering their world vicariously, I got lost in it enough to temporarily forget my own tension about where I was and what I was doing.

One song played over and over on the jukebox, like an anthem. I was struck with the irony of the lyrics:

It's a big wide wonderful world we live in.
When you're in love you're a hero,
a Nero, a wizard, a gay Santa Claus.

The world of Terry's Bar felt not big and wide but small and narrow; the people around me felt not like heroes but casualties. Maybe hearing those lyrics over and over worked a kind of magic, created an illusion that homosexual love could be transforming, but I didn't believe it and I doubted if these women really did either.

I began to wonder what I had been so afraid would happen to me in this place. The women there didn't seem interested in me. Was I safe from them? Did I want to be? Was I more afraid of what might stir within me than in any of them, what demons I would be unable to control? I didn't know what to think, but I was sure of one thing—I had crossed over a line and found on the other side not the peril I had imagined but a profound curiosity.

The next day I told Marilyn that I understood why Rusty didn't wear lipstick and why it was *always* ladies night at Terry's Bar, that she didn't have to pretend with me because I had been thinking for some time that I might be homosexual, too. The word came out in a hoarse whisper. Did I really say that out loud? Marilyn looked very interested.

"Well, I'm not sure I am, but I might be," I went on. "I mean I've been attracted to women, I'm attracted to men too, but not in the same way, not exactly, I mean, I'm attracted to *both*." Marilyn was smiling. "I'm glad you told me."

"I'm glad too. I came to New York to find out, you know, if I am. It's hard to be sure if you've never . . . well, you know what I mean."

"Yes, I know," Marilyn said.

I had just revealed myself to a person I'd known two days. I felt an enormous sense of relief, released for a moment from the burden of the secret by saying those words aloud.

I became a regular at Terry's Bar, usually going there with Marilyn and her friends. Even when I went alone no one paid attention to me, and I was too shy to approach anybody. Mostly I listened.

47

A great many of the women at Terry's were estranged from their families or deeply into a charade of pretending they were career-minded bachelor girls, just waiting for the right man, or attached to a boyfriend (who was really a gay man who could "pass" and was willing to play the game). They were all in the closet with the door firmly nailed shut. Subterfuge and deception marked their passage through a homosexual-hating world.

In 1950 discrimination against homosexuals was so pervasive in the society that anger about it had no identifiable target, whatever rage there was turned in on itself and became a toxic force, a spoiler of love and a killer of dreams. Why didn't they protest? There was no concept of gay activism or liberation then. Silence and invisibility were the only reliable strategies, and seemingly always would be. These women sat huddled together in a smoke-filled bar that was their haven. Here they played out the never-ending intrigues of their tangled love lives. Romance was the palliative that softened despair, that made it all bearable.

I was rarely bored at Terry's Bar. Several of the women had movie-star fathers, and they loved to tell deglamourizing stories about their parents, payback perhaps for the outcast role they were afforded in their families. One regular's father was a well-known philosopher who had just written a book that was the talk of intellectual America.

These women were interesting in their own way, but the queen bee was my roommate Marilyn. She was the elusive beauty who kept everyone infatuated and dangling on the hook. I was as attracted to her as the others, but she didn't even flirt with me. I wasn't surprised. Why would anyone as glamorous and popular as she was be romantically interested in me?

One night I was alone with the philosopher's daughter. As we talked I noticed that she was moving closer to me. I felt an immediate rush. At last something was going to happen. She leaned forward and kissed me on the mouth. I closed my eyes and gave myself over to the feelings, melting inside, excited to have this contact at last. Then, suddenly, she was saying something: "I don't think this is a good idea."

I couldn't believe it. What did I do wrong? "Why is it not a good idea?" She paused, then admitted, "Marilyn wouldn't like it."

I got it. The queen bee had warned all her loyal subjects to stay away from me. As long as I was paying Marilyn's rent, I was off limits to her friends, the untouchable ingenue with a job. That did it. No, that didn't quite do it. Two subsequent events did.

One night I was in bed asleep. Marilyn came in and she had someone with her, which hadn't happened before. Her studio couch was about three feet from mine, so I heard her whisper, "It's okay. She's asleep." Of course, I was never more wide awake. I shut my eyes tight. I saw nothing but I heard everything. First there were murmurings, giggles, much moving about, then groans, more moving about, heavy breathing, more groans. It went on for what seemed like hours. I tried to shut out what was happening, but that was impossible. I felt trapped, playing dead, scared of making a sound, near tears. Finally, it was over, some muffled talk, and the visitor went to the bathroom. When she came out, she dressed and left. I had no idea who the visitor was and I didn't want to know.

In the morning, Marilyn behaved as though nothing unusual had happened the night before, but I could think of nothing else. I didn't know what to say. I felt, in turn, angry, embarrassed, stupid, and hurt. I wasn't sure I had a right to feel angry or hurt, but I was definitely embarrassed and felt stupid that I was so dumb about what to say. I convinced myself that either Marilyn would deny that anything happened, or she simply wouldn't give a damn about my feelings. I felt defeated. I chose silence.

The second event was another humiliation, this one so traumatic I couldn't ignore it. Marilyn threw a party in our apartment. It was an extraordinary affair, the gang from Terry's Bar was invited plus some women I'd never seen before, some stylishly feminine, others stylishly masculine. The room was very crowded and, as always happens with short people at stand-up parties, I got bumped, elbowed, and spilled on. To protect myself, I retreated to the edge of the crowd and propped myself against the wall. The music from the phonograph blared out at full volume. Smoke hung in the air. As the wine flowed, the din of conversation began to compete with the music.

Suddenly, something startling happened. As if by a signal, the entire room lapsed into silence. All eyes turned to one corner where a woman stood alone. Slowly she began to sing, without accompaniment. Her voice was honey sweet, mellow and melodic, soothing. She sang to the hushed room. I didn't know who she was, but I found her enchanting. When the song was completed, everyone shouted for an encore. She sang again, and when she finished, she bowed to thunderous applause and moved immediately back into the crowd. I turned to a woman standing next to me and asked, "Who was that?"

"Honey, you don't know who that was? That was the one and only Mabel Mercer. You just had a real special treat."

49

I didn't realize at the time how special it was to witness Mabel Mercer performing at a party. I just knew I was warmed inside by her singing. After Mabel sang, the sound level in the room rose rapidly. I spent the next hour wandering around the party, standing on the edge of conversations, trying to find a way to participate. I drank to dull the pain I was beginning to feel as the perpetual outsider. Why was it so easy for me to relate to men and so difficult to connect with women? What was wrong with me?

Exhausted and drunk, I sank into a chair. I was staring into space, feeling sorry for myself when it happened. I've never figured out why it happened, or who did it, or what it was supposed to mean, but someone standing behind me suddenly emptied an enormous ashtray, brimming over with ashes and cigarette butts, onto my head. I sat there stunned, ashes dripping off my face, cigarette butts in my hair. Several people rushed to my side and began brushing the mess off me. I couldn't move. I felt like someone who had just tumbled down the stairs, then felt embarrassed about causing a problem. I wanted to scream but I couldn't even cry. I just sat dead still.

The philosopher's daughter was leaning over me. She put her face very close to mine, looked directly into my eyes, and spoke in a quiet, firm voice, "You know, this is not the place for you. You're too nice and too young and you're not ready for this. Go home." Her words penetrated the haze in my brain. I knew she was right. I left New York the next day.

The year is 1985. Thirty-five years later, I am returning to MacDougal Street looking for Terry's Bar. What I find in that exact spot is the New York University Law School. I look up the philosopher's daughter. She receives me but is not too interested in my visit. I ask her what I was like back then.

"You were a scared little rabbit," she says.

She describes some of my behavior, and I don't like hearing it. I want to interrupt her, to say that I'm not scared any more. I am a confident, mature person, a psychotherapist, an author, an activist working to make the lives of gay and lesbian people better. I want to tell this to all the MacDougal Street lesbians who didn't give the time of day to the scared little rabbit. I want to shout into the past, to amend the record, to redeem myself, but I know it will do no good. They won't hear me because there isn't anybody there anymore.

5

In a move that had to come from the healthier part of my being, I went from New York to St. Louis seeking the healing experience I knew I would have in the home of Aunt Rose, my father's older sister and the matriarch of the family. She asked no questions, fattened me up on her Jewish cooking, and gave me loving attention. She had two sons but had always wanted a daughter. I was lucky enough to be that surrogate for the next few months.

At Aunt Rose's I stayed in the room that had belonged to her sons, memorabilia of an untroubled adolescence all over the place—high school pennants, a small portable phonograph on a record cabinet holding orderly rows of 78s, silver-backed military hair brushes neatly lined up atop a polished-pine chest of drawers. In this setting my world began to feel right-side up again. I got a job working at Hagedorn's Bookstore in downtown St. Louis. I spent my evenings with old friends from childhood or visiting with Aunt Rose and Uncle Leon, listening to the radio, or going for rides in Leon's car. I felt very safe and that was enough for a while, but the call of adventure soon began to stir in me again.

I had heard that Jay Landesman, the editor of an avant-garde magazine called *Neurotica*, was living in St. Louis. I called him and we became fast friends. I talked to Jay about my sexual confusion, my failed attempts to be a lesbian, my uncertainly about what to do next. Jay said he thought I needed professional help, and he referred me to his psychiatrist who was willing to see me "after hours" at a reduced fee. I have come to think of this therapist as Dr. Strangebird.

Dr. Strangebird was a fat little man whose glasses were continually sliding down his tiny nose, to be pushed up again by a pudgy finger. On our first visit he motioned me to a chair, loosened his tie, stretched out on his couch, and lit a very large cigar.

"So tell me about yourself."

I'd never been in therapy before, but I'd been to the movies and seen a lot of *New Yorker* cartoons, and I knew there was something wrong with this picture: therapist on the couch, patient in the chair. Because I was getting a discounted fee, I thought maybe I didn't rate the couch. Nevertheless, I was there to talk about myself, and talk I did, week after week, pouring out the conflict and confusion that I felt about myself.

Dr. Strangebird had little to say, grunts, "hmmmm," and "I see." I felt like I was in an echo chamber, but it didn't matter because I was discovering that I was good at seeing the patterns in my own behavior. I felt helped by the opportunity to talk through thoughts and feelings that had been all jumbled up inside me.

After a dozen sessions I thought I'd gone as far as I could go in the echo chamber of Dr. Strangebird's office. When I announced that I was not coming back anymore, Dr. Strangebird lifted himself with his usual difficulty off the couch, held out a beefy hand, and said, "So, good luck, my dear. It's been a pleasure to know you." Had it? How could I tell? Still, since I didn't know any better, I assumed this was the way it was done.

When I think back on it now, my mind is boggled by this doctor's bizarre conduct, puffing away at his cigar, either staring at the ceiling or checking his watch. What was he doing? To this day I'm clueless. When a patient announces precipitously that she is not returning, it usually means something is not going right in the therapy relationship: "You aren't listening to me. You don't care about me. Pay attention to me." No such interpretations from Dr. Strangebird, just a cheerful good-bye and a wave out the door. It didn't matter. I'd had enough of ruminating anyway. I was ready to get on with life, my self-esteem considerably shored up by Aunt Rose's loving care.

I left St. Louis in high spirits, headed for California to finish my education. My reason for stopping in Tucson was to see Barbara, my best friend from high school who had just had her first baby. My reason for looking up the two lesbians in Tucson who were friends of the MacDougal Street crowd was that I was bored after a few days with Barbara and her husband. I was also resentful that Barbara had such a fulfilling life while I was still trying to figure out who and what I was.

I was nervous about making the phone call. I knew I shouldn't, the Mac-Dougal Street lesbians had not been kind to me, but somehow they still intrigued me, plus I needed to get away from the cloying "normalcy" of Barbara's life, my envy of it, my anger about it, and my inability to reconcile these feelings.

"Come on over," Luce said.

In ten minutes I was in the living room of Lila and Luce's sun-washed desert adobe house. Lila was thin and fragile looking, the one in Tucson for her health. Her eyes had a penetrating quality that went with her intense, deliberate way of speaking in a voice too deep for such a small person. Luce was tall, slim, and boyishly handsome, a Spanish aristocrat with dark, luminous eyes and raven-black hair. I liked them both immediately.

They were eager for New York gossip even though mine was months old. I did not touch on my own tribulations with the MacDougal Street crowd. I just repeated what I had heard as the fly on the wall in Terry's Bar. I was surprised when I realized it was getting dark. Barbara would wonder where I was. I didn't know how I would explain my absence—visiting with a couple of dykes from New York because I was bored with her family scene. Lila and Luce begged me to come back the next day. I told them I had to get on to Los Angeles.

"No, no," they protested. "Come stay here with us. We have plenty of room."

This hospitality was quite different from the way I had been treated by the New York lesbians. I was flattered and I agreed. The next day Barbara took me to the train. I hoisted my bags into the vestibule, then climbed on board waving Barbara off with the assurance that I would be fine. The minute she was out of sight, I swung off the other side of the train where Lila and Luce were waiting.

Titillated by pulling off our little deception, we began a two-week adventure, accompanied by Luce and Lila's gay male friend, Brook, a displaced easterner with an elegant French poodle named Louie. Brook had a shiny black jeep in which we careened around the desert, a merry quartet, blithe spirits forming ties that would bind our lives together in ways we couldn't have imagined then.

The adventure came to a halt when Lila left on a trip to visit her family in Ohio. For some reason she had to fly out of Albuquerque, so the four of us drove all day from Tucson. We waved Lila off and checked into a hotel, Luce and I sharing a room. As we dressed to go out for dinner, I watched Luce, lean and elegant, and I felt something stirring in me. How could I have such feelings? Lila had been so good to me. How could I even think of betraying her trust?

After dinner we drove to an old western bar we'd passed on the way from the airport. We imagined a lively scene inside, cowboys and their ladies dancing to country tunes. We pushed through the swinging doors and stopped dead in our tracks. The barnlike interior was empty, still, silent. A few grizzled old men sat on bar stools, unmoving, staring straight ahead. The bartender waved us toward the empty tables. Overhead, a cut-glass ball revolved ever so slowly, playing circles of light on the deserted dance floor. Brook brought two pitchers of beer to the table. We fed the jukebox and the room was suddenly filled with the sounds of hearty hoe-down music. Swilling the beer, we were soon up and dancing, the three of us, arms linked, twirling around the dance floor, giggling, going faster and faster until Brook screamed, "Stop, I can't do it anymore. I'm dizzy!" and we all fell into chairs enervated and out of breath. I guess we were too much for the old guys at the bar because every one of them was gone. The bartender didn't seem to mind us though, probably a welcome relief from his usual taciturn crew. He brought another pitcher of beer, which we injudiciously chugalugged.

It was about then that I peered into the darkness at the back of the room and saw the bicycle leaning against the wall. Was it really a bicycle or was I imagining it? I got up and went to investigate. It was real and obviously there for me to ride, so I wheeled it onto the dance floor and climbed on. I pedaled steadily at first, round and round, picking up speed until I was sailing through the air on a magical mystery ride, being pedaled through Forest Park by my father, my mother alongside, the breeze in my face, every-thing right with the world. I felt blissful, cared for, attended to, protected, a child needing only to be a child as I went round and round, but the good feelings soon slipped away and I was a lost child, alone, frightened, running away from myself, not knowing how to stop the dizzying circles, crying, crying for help. I came to a stop in the middle of the dance floor and just sat there bewildered.

In slow motion, Luce and Brook were coming toward me. They lifted me off the bicycle and held me between them without saying a word. Once again I was taken care of. Brook went to settle up with the bartender while Luce carefully guided me through the swinging doors. I don't remember anything after that until I woke up in the hotel room. Luce's arms were around me. She smiled as I opened my eyes.

"Okay?" she asked.

"Okay." With that she got up and moved to the other bed. The next day we drove back to Tucson.

In the days ahead I knew I was in trouble because I could think of nothing but Luce. I couldn't get her out of my mind; I wanted to feel her next to me again, her face close to mine. I would become so overwhelmed by these feelings I'd have to stop what I was doing and give myself over to the reverie. I was lost. I had no idea whether she had feelings for me. Was this just my fantasy? What could I say to her? What if she didn't take me seriously, laughed at me, rejected me? I didn't know what to do.

"I'll take those," Luce said as I appeared in the laundry room of the house with an armful of clothes. I watched her stuff my things into the washing machine and twirl the dials. I was frozen in place, too scared to speak, the awkward teenager trapped inside myself, immobilized by shyness.

Luce was smiling as she approached me, putting her arms around me, drawing me to her, kissing me. I could feel that kiss shoot throughout my body. I'd never felt anything like it before. Our mouths were still pressed together as she lowered me to the floor. Her body was on top of mine, then mine on hers as we rolled over and over. I could feel a momentum building inside me with such force I thought I would explode. I was going out of control, and when the feelings became unbearable I let out a scream that seemed to cue all the vibrations inside me to a violent climax. I didn't want to think, only to feel, but the realization that I had just had my first orgasm with another human being played over and over in my head like a needle stuck in the groove of a record. I felt ecstatic.

The next two weeks were pure bliss. We hardly left the house, hardly left the bed. I floated through the days, oblivious to everything but what was happening with Luce. When she left me to go to another room, I could hardly stand it until she came back. For the first time in my life I was in love, and sure I was loved in return.

Then the bubble burst. Lila was coming home. Decisions had to be made. Luce had been trying to talk to me for some time about her relationship with Lila, but I hadn't wanted to hear it. Now there was no choice. I had to listen to her feelings of ambivalence about Lila. I had to hear about the dilemma she was faced with and how difficult the decision was going to be for her. I told her that there was only one decision possible—that she and I would be together. It simply had to be that way. I was startled at my own assertiveness, but I was not going to let go of this extraordinary experience of being in love, not now, not ever.

As the day of Lila's homecoming neared, we decided it would be best for me to be gone when she arrived. Luce's plan was to tell Lila what had happened, stay around for a few days to deal with Lila's reaction, then say she was going to visit me in California to sort out her feelings. With great reluctance I left. The train ride from Tucson to Los Angeles seemed interminable. What I was doing felt crazy. All I wanted was to be with Luce, but with every passing minute I found myself further and further away from her.

My mother was distraught, not because I had disappeared and Barbara was calling every day to see if I'd gotten home, but because my father had left her for another woman.

"How long has this been going on?" I asked foolishly, since I knew that my father had been cheating for decades.

"What do you care? You're no help to me. I had no idea where you were and at this point I don't care. I'd just as soon you were out of this house for good!"

I understood my mother's anger, but for a moment the old fear came back—she was displeased, was she going to abandon me? I realized that it no longer mattered. I had already abandoned her. What I needed now was practical support. I was out of money and had no place to live. I had to call my father. I couldn't think of anything else to do.

I had mixed feelings about my father. His infidelity and my mother's misery over it had been the dominant themes of my adolescence. I'd hated him for what he did to our family, and my mother encouraged me to hate him. It was the bond between us—being angry at him was my way to stay in her favor. On the other hand, I admired my father's ability to do whatever he pleased and get away with it. If there was a parent to model myself after, he was it. He seemed to get more out of life than she did. Being angry at him seemed pointless now. It didn't even earn me my mother's approval anymore.

The one thing I most regretted about being banished from my mother's house was the lost opportunity to see much of my little sister. She was twelve then and at the beginning of what would become an absorbing theatrical career. I had neglected her in my preoccupation with figuring out what I was all about. Now my own problems continued to absorb me, and I wouldn't really get to know her until much later in our lives.

When my father told me about the woman he was having a relationship with, Mrs. Green, I reminded myself that I didn't have to be angry. Here was a whole new scenario. I was no longer lobbying for my mother's affection. I didn't have to be angry at all. He said he was going to marry Mrs. Green (what I have always called her) and live in her house in Brentwood, so I could have the little apartment he was then living in. He peeled off a few $100 bills from the wad he customarily carried and put them in my hand.

I decided I had better tell him about Luce because he would have to know sooner or later. As I began, I realized I would also be telling him that I was homosexual, which I was not prepared to hear myself say to him quite yet. Why was it so difficult to say that I loved someone? My head was spinning. What was I doing to myself? I just blurted it out: "Dad, this might be a good time to tell you that I'm involved with someone, too. It's a woman." As soon as I said the words, I wanted to take them back, but it was too late.

He looked at me in disbelief. "Are you sure about this?" he asked.

"I don't know. I think so."

"I think you're all mixed up."

"I probably am."

"What are you going to do?"

"About what?"

"This problem."

"Which one?"

"This woman."

"I hope she's going to come here and live with me."

He looked at me for a long time before he spoke. "Okay, if that's the way it is, that's the way it is."

I couldn't believe he was accepting this so easily. Perhaps he recognized that his own life was anything but exemplary, or maybe it was just not worth the trouble to be in conflict with me. As a father, he had always taken the easy way out. This time it worked to my advantage. I knew that he was going to be on my side and I didn't care why. I needed him.

A week later Luce arrived. A week after that Lila arrived. Were we going to be one big unhappy family? I was afraid that I was going to have to compete with Lila, whom I saw as smarter and more sophisticated than I. She knew her way around as a lesbian and she had a history with Luce. I, on the other hand, was new to the game, and I felt nervous at the thought of fighting for Luce. One thing was certain: our idyll in the desert was over.

Luce spent her time shuttling between Lila and me, which only increased my insecurity. Whenever Lila called, Luce flew to her side, and each time I resented it. I decided that I had to find a way to integrate myself into the relationship of these two women. With some trepidation, I set up an evening with Lila, who I had not seen since waving her off at the Albuquerque airport. She was cool but cordial to me.

"I would like us to be friends," I began.

Lila looked at me as though I were crazy. "I don't know if that's possible," she responded.

"I know you're angry, and I don't blame you. It was not something I planned. I'm terribly sorry you were hurt. I really like and admire you," and as I said it, I realized how true it was. I'd fallen in love with Luce, but I was drawn to Lila's quick mind and intellectual intensity. The sincerity of my feelings must have come through.

"Well, I suppose there's nothing to be gained by being at war with you. I'll try to be friends, but I'm wary of you."

"I understand."

"I don't forgive you."

"That's all right."

"I can't believe I'm doing this."

"You won't be sorry."

I truly wanted to be in Lila's good graces again, and in that moment I flashed on a familiar experience—begging my mother's forgiveness for some childhood transgression, desperate for the reassurance that I was still okay with her.

My campaign with Lila worked. She allowed a friendship to develop again and it made my relationship with Luce much less tense. As that problem eased, I had to face the emergence of another one, the resurfacing of my old conflict about being a homosexual.

There were times when I wanted to reject altogether the reality of being a lesbian. I hated that word. It made me want to push Luce away. The problem was that I also loved her and wanted to be close to her, forever.

To further complicate my feelings, I was beginning to see troubling aspects of Luce's personality. She seemed to have an aversion to earning a living. Raised in the aristocratic tradition of an early California Spanish land-grant family, she was not trained for the world of work, but the family's fortune had run out and with it the support she was accustomed to. Without a work history Luce could only find jobs that were beneath her intelligence and level of sophistication, so of course she didn't want to work. Lila apparently had family money to take care of that issue. I had only what I could earn, and it scared me to think about supporting another person, but there seemed to be no choice. I had to find a job. I was in a steep learning curve about the practicalities of a real-world relationship.

Bennett and Marshall, Booksellers, had a magnificent stock of rare books, prints, and maps dating back to the fourteenth century. They also carried out-of-print contemporary books. Their help wanted ad asked for an "experienced cataloger of antiquarian books." I answered their questions at the interview with as much honesty as I could muster, which wasn't much: "Yes, I've worked in bookstores all over the country." "Yes, I can catalog antiquarian books." (Not sure what that even meant.) "No, I don't know anything about old prints and maps, but I can learn." (I hoped.)

They bought it all and hired me. I went directly from their store to the public library where I checked out a stack of books on illuminated manuscripts, and incunabula (which I learned were books printed before 1501). I studied hard, immersing myself in the esoterica of rare books and prints from the sixteenth to the twentieth centuries.

At work, I pored over auction records and other booksellers' catalogs until I thought I could put together a passable catalog of my own. My first attempt, "Seven Centuries: 14th to 20th Inclusive," won high praise from university librarians and collectors. I could relax. At twenty-two I became the youngest member of the venerable Antiquarian Booksellers Association of America.

I loved working in the past. Some years later I tried to get hired as a librarian at the William Andrews Clark Library, part of the UCLA system. The Clark Library had manuscripts that were so old and precious they were kept under lock and key, and could only be perused by scholars under the watchful eye of a guard. Lawrence Clark Powell was a dear, sweet man, then head librarian of UCLA (today his name is carved in stone above the entrance to UCLA's main library). He responded to my job application in person because I knew him from my work at Bennett and Marshall.

"Betty, I wouldn't dare give you this job. You're too bright and alive to bury yourself in the antiquities. Get out of here and go do something in the world of today!"

What a favor he did me.

My father had by then married Mrs. Green, and Luce and I were frequent dinner guests in her home. Mrs. Green was a successful businesswoman, an attractive, chic, gracious person who seemed quite comfortable with my relationship with Luce. One night at dinner I spoke about a dream I had— to have my own bookstore, selling avant-garde books, the Frances Steloff of the West. Almost immediately I felt foolish talking about running a business at my age, but Mrs. Green didn't think it was foolish at all. When she called me the next morning with an offer to back me in opening my own store, I nearly fell off my chair.

My father assured me that she was serious and could well afford the $10,000 she deposited in a bank account for me. I was in shock. What if I failed? Mrs. Green said that I shouldn't be thinking about failure before I even tried and that the money was not a loan but a gift, so there was nothing to lose.

I started to think about everything that could go wrong. I told myself to shut up, stop anticipating disaster. I'd worked in five bookstores by then, I'd accompanied Bennett and Marshall on book buys. I knew a lot about publishers, acquiring out-of-print books, cataloging, selling to the public. I could do this. Allow the dream. Accept the gift. Do it.

6

On November 1, 1950, I opened the doors to Berzon Books on Las Palmas, half a block off the busiest part of Hollywood Boulevard. The shelves were in, permits obtained, signs up, ads taken, books bought, window dressed, and art hung in the gallery space above the bookshelves. I could hardly believe it was actually happening, but when I sold my first book on November 2, I knew it was for real.

Business came with the foot traffic from the Las Palmas Theater across the street and the twenty-four-hour newsstand two doors away. I turned the back of the store into a kind of salon where people gathered to drink tea and coffee and talk of things literary. When I wasn't feeling like Frances Steloff, I was feeling like Gertrude Stein.

Luce worked in the store with me, but she spent most evenings socializing in the back until ten o'clock, when I closed up and we all adjourned to the House of Ivy bar across the street. It never occurred to me to question the pace of my life; I opened at ten in the morning and closed twelve hours later, six days a week. I had boundless energy and a sense of mission that kept it all moving and exciting.

The notice in *Publisher's Weekly* said that Dr. Edith Sitwell (three years later Dame Edith) and her brother, Sir Osbert, were going to pay their first visit to the West Coast of the United States in January. I immediately began to daydream—what an opening event that would be, a party for the Sitwells, the premier literary family of England. In the dream, they would come to my store for a reception, hundreds of people would attend, and I would become famous for hosting Dr. Edith and Sir Osbert on their first trip to Los Angeles.

What a fantasy! What nonsense! Was I crazy? What publisher would allow *me* to do that? But I couldn't let go of the dream. What harm was there in trying? I wrote to Vanguard Press, Edith Sitwell's publisher, and to my astonishment they wrote back saying, yes, I could host a reception on the morning of January 9, the Sitwells had other plans for the rest of the day. Was I dreaming? I read the letter twenty times. It was all part of the miracle—I owned a bookstore and I was giving a party for two of the most famous people in the literary world. I giggled at myself. What next?

The first thing I heard was that Louie Epstein, owner of the Pickwick Bookstore, was in a fury. The Pickwick, around the corner on Hollywood Boulevard, was the largest and most prestigious bookstore on the West Coast. Louie's letter to Vanguard arrived after mine. They were honoring their commitment to me. He'd called them to say that I was just a young girl with a tiny new bookstore that hardly had any books in it, that it would be ludicrous to let me host the Sitwells, but Vanguard stood their ground. I was amazed and panicked.

I took an ad in the *Los Angeles Times* and sent press releases everywhere. I mailed five hundred invitations to Bennett and Marshall's mailing list, which I'd shamelessly purloined. I went to a theatrical prop house and rented two thrones and a red carpet, and I hired a photographer to record the monumental event. Then came a glitch. Edith never allowed herself to be photographed before noon. "Don't worry," my photographer said. "I will take pictures and she'll never know there is a camera in the room." He did. I saw him behind bookcases and under tables, no flash. She never saw him at all and I ended up with photographs to treasure.

My ad in the in the *Los Angeles Times* read:

Berzon Books cordially invites you to a Breakfast Party for Dr. Edith and Sir Osbert Sitwell, 10 A.M., Tuesday, January 9th, 1645 North Las Palmas, Hollywood. No charge.

Then I worried that no one would come to a morning event. I imagined six people there, and I would not only be embarrassed but ruined. I fretted about something different every chance I had.

The day arrived. I'd borrowed my father's car and recruited Bill, an actor friend with a fake British accent, to chauffeur me to the Bel Air Hotel to pick up the Sitwells. I was a nervous wreck. As we drove along Sunset Boulevard toward the hotel, I felt as though I were going to the guillotine.

"Okay, I can do this," I kept telling myself over and over. "I can do this."

Bill stayed in the car while I went into the lobby to call the Sitwells. They were already there, waiting.

"You must be Miss Berzon," Edith Sitwell said as she rose from her chair. She seemed to endlessly unfold herself until she stood towering over me, all six feet three inches of her. Her height was spectacular enough but her costume was even more so. She wore a full-length velvet coat over a floor-length velvet dress. Although it was seventy-five degrees outside, her hands were encased in fur-trimmed velvet gloves that came almost to her elbows. The entire outfit was topped off by a velvet artist's palette hat that swept across one side of her head.

I was speechless. Still more startling than her outfit was her face. It was unusually long and white, a veritable beak of a nose sprouting at its center. Just above the beak were two narrow slits of pink-rimmed eyes that narrowed even more as the thin red line of her mouth smiled.

"Dr. Sitwell," I managed. "I'm so pleased to meet you."

Out of the corner of my eye I saw Sir Osbert struggling to rise from his chair. His presentation was not so dramatic as his sister's. The most noticeable thing about him was the palsied shaking of his hands. He nodded in my direction and mumbled something that sounded like "Good morning." We headed for the door.

Edith and I shared the back seat, where she chatted amiably, but when she addressed me, she did not turn her face toward me, perhaps because of the wide swing of her hat. Instead, she inclined her entire body sideways in my direction. This necessitated addressing her in profile, for which I was grateful, for looking fully into those pink little eyes was very disconcerting.

Edith constantly commented on the greenery she saw along the way, calling Osbert's attention particularly to the mimosa. Bill engaged Osbert in short bursts of conversation that sounded more like throat clearings than language. It seemed to be going okay, but I was preoccupied with what we would find when we arrived at the bookstore.

As the car turned into Hollywood Boulevard and neared Las Palmas I could see that there was some sort of commotion in the street. "Oh, no!" I thought. "There's been a disaster—a car crash, a murder, a fire!" A motorcycle cop held up his hand to stop us at the corner of Hollywood Boulevard and Las Palmas. As we pulled up to him I could see that the entire block of Las Palmas was filled with people. Bill asked what was happening.

"There's some sort of party in a bookstore down there and so many people showed up we had to close off the street."

I thought I was going to faint. Bill informed the officer that we were delivering the guests of honor to the party. The cop peered into the car and upon seeing the apparition in velvet in the backseat he immediately waved us through. We inched toward the curb and stopped. As the Sitwells alighted

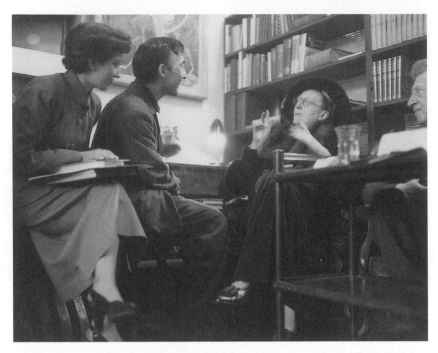

The Berzon Books reception for Edith and Osbert Sitwell, where I nervously
monitored Samson DeBrier's conversation with Dr. Edith about why she didn't
open her door to him when he was a young student in London.

from the car and made their way over the red carpet, a hush came over the
crowd. Inside, the bookstore was jammed with people. As I led the Sitwells
along, ever so slowly, a voice drifted up from the crowd.

"Wait 'til the Bel Air finds out what she did with their drapes!"

I dared not look at the Sitwells.

Once I had Edith and Osbert seated on their thrones, I placed a small
tea cart before them on which I'd put glasses of water and fountain pens.
I positioned two chairs in front of the cart. The crowd was well behaved,
waiting patiently in line to have their books signed, leaning over on the way
to help themselves to coffee and danish as they passed the "breakfast" table.

It was going okay when suddenly I noticed the person about to sit down
in front of the Sitwells. It was Samson DeBrier, whom the *Los Angeles Times*
called "the longest established eccentric this side of the Sierra." My warning
signals went off. Samson was a well-known character on the Hollywood
fringe, particularly famous for his exotic parties and the outlandish costumes
he wore to them, often changing at least three times an evening. Samson

was a friend, a sweet man, but unpredictable. He seemed a little agitated as he seated himself in front of Edith Sitwell. I slipped into the chair next to him.

Samson began, "Dr. Sitwell, some years ago when I was a poor student living in London, I called on you. I came to your flat. You answered my knock, but you would not open your door to me. I was quite offended. I only wanted to talk about your poetry, of which I was an ardent fan. I meant no harm. Please tell me, why didn't you open your door to me?"

Edith Sitwell looked pensive. "Just when was that, my dear?" she asked.

Samson told her the year and she nodded thoughtfully.

"Oh yes, I remember now. That was the year there was a series of grisly murders in London and the police instructed us never to open our door to anyone we didn't know."

Samson looked dubious. Edith Sitwell leaned forward and spoke in a sincere whisper, "My dear, if you are ever in London again, I hope you will call on me and I will *certainly* open my door to you this time." She gave his hand a dismissive pat and smiled him on his way as the next person approached. I breathed a sigh of relief.

After a little more than an hour, I could see the Sitwells were growing weary. I suggested it was time to leave and they both looked appreciative. We made our way slowly back through the crowd. Edith smiled and waved the queenly wave. Osbert seemed intent only on reaching the door.

In the car, Edith settled into the back seat and began to debrief the party. "Osbert, there was this odd man who came to see me in London when he was a student. He said he was offended because I wouldn't open my door to him. Well, I don't remember that, of course, but I made up a story about grisly murders and the police warning us not to open our doors to strangers. He seemed satisfied with that. Oh, Osbert, look at the mimosa! Isn't it beautiful?" Osbert nodded and mumbled something unintelligible.

Edith leaned back and lapsed into silence. She seemed to be enjoying some private thought. I watched her carefully, wondering what other stories she was preparing to regale Osbert with once they were alone. I began to feel a little nervous about the absence of conversation, then I remembered having seen an interview in which Edith Sitwell was asked what her favorite recreation was. She had replied, "Silence." She did not speak again until we pulled into the driveway of the Bel Air Hotel.

"This has been most enjoyable, my dear. Thank you so much for arranging it," she said, leaning sideways to me.

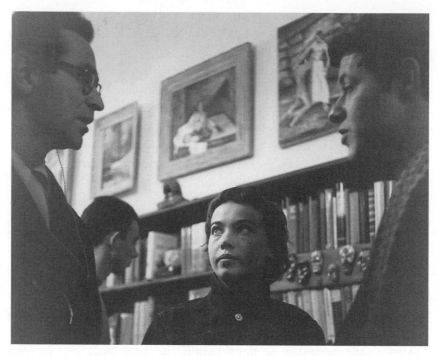

One of the events at Berzon Books. Dahn Ben-Amotz, on the right, later became a
celebrated writer and filmmaker in Israel. His friend, Leslie Carron, a young
French dancer, was in town to film *An American in Paris*.

As Bill came around to the passenger side to throw open the front and
back doors, Edith leaned toward me and extended her hand. I grasped the
long, bony fingers and held them for a few seconds, feeling a little unreal
holding Edith Sitwell's hand. Then she slipped her fingers away and was out
of the car, smiling, waving, and disappearing up the path to the hotel, Osbert
following tremulously a few steps behind her.

I felt exuberant. I had actually pulled it off. I threw myself back on the
frontseat feeling as though tons of weight had been lifted from me. I babbled
to Bill all the way back to the bookstore.

The Sitwell party established Berzon Books as a presence on the Los
Angeles literary scene. One newspaper reported:

The Berzon Book Store in Hollywood is swiftly becoming the hangout of the "avant-gardist." Not long ago Miss Berzon held a breakfast
party for the English poets, the Sitwells, then she had Anaïs Nin recite
some of her poetry, and last Sunday night she showed two experimen-

tal films, Ian Hugo's *Ai-Ye* (Mankind) and Sam Zebba's *Uriapuru* (Bird of Love). Poetess Anaïs Nin discussed the films after the showing.

Anaïs Nin came into my life through Lila, who had known her in New York. To say merely that Anaïs was a complex individual would greatly understate the case. Her fragile beauty compelled the eye. The richness of her language and the soft accents of her voice commanded the listener's attention. There was a certain power in her presence, despite the fact, or perhaps because of it, that just below the surface you could always sense her vulnerability, making her seem like someone who needed your protection even as she was overpowering you.

In 1951 Anaïs was a cult figure in the literary world just beginning to be commercially published and critically acknowledged. Because she was living in Los Angeles at the time, she decided to make my bookstore her headquarters, using it as her mailing address and giving me fine editions of her early work on consignment, many printed on her own handpress.

When I put out my first catalog, Anaïs wrote the introduction:

The world of art in America is dissociated. Whoever makes for us a selection of values in books, paintings, people, is contributing vitally to its integration and therefore to its strength. Betty Berzon is doing this for us in Hollywood, with both good taste and human friendliness.

I was very moved by her words, and I presented Anaïs in a reading of her poetry to a standing-room-only crowd. Soon I became known as the official purveyor of the works of Anaïs Nin. Our relationship grew as Luce and I spent evenings with her and her husband, Rupert Pole, who was a U.S. forest ranger at the time. He and Anaïs lived at the ranger station in Sierra Madre, a remote forest town and a singularly incongruent habitat for exotic, worldly, delicate Anaïs. Rupert was no ordinary forest ranger. He was an accomplished cellist, a former actor, and a man of dazzling good looks.

A week after Anaïs's reading I scheduled the showing of two avant-garde films; Anaïs, who knew both filmmakers, led the discussion. What I did not know was that Anaïs was also married to filmmaker Ian Hugo, who was actually an international banker named Hugo Guiler. I soon learned that it was an ill-kept secret that Anaïs was legally married to two men at once, Rupert in Los Angeles and Hugo in New York. She split her time between them telling Rupert that she was committed to spend six months each year working for Fleur Cowles at the New York offices of her magazine, *Fleur*. I don't know what she told Hugo.

Rupert's mother was married to Frank Lloyd Wright's son, Lloyd Wright, himself a prominent architect. The Wright family gathered weekly in West Hollywood at the great stone mansion of the paterfamilias to play music. I knew about the gatherings because my cousin, Ronald Stein, a musician and film composer, was a regular at these Wright family musicales. I thought about Anaïs and what a welcome respite these evenings must have been from her life in the forest. Her other respite, I assume, was her "Fleur Cowles job" in New York.

It was during one of Anaïs's New York trips that Rupert came into the bookstore and rewrote the scenario of our friendship. Late in the evening, Luce was in the back with the coffee klatch. Rupert said he came by because he was feeling lonely. I was appropriately sympathetic, somehow not noticing that he was standing very close to me. I certainly did notice when he leaned over and kissed me. I was shocked, but captivated. I didn't know what to say, but before I could even think about that, Rupert swooped me up and threw me over his shoulder in a fireman's carry. I squealed, which brought Luce out front, stopping dead in her tracks at the sight of me being carried toward the front door. "She'll be back tomorrow," Rupert shouted, laughing and twirling me around as we left the bookstore.

Incredible as it seems now, I didn't object, and Luce didn't have time to. Did Rupert give a thought to the fact that I was in a relationship that should be as sacred as a marriage? No, but then I didn't give that a thought either. I was flattered and excited by Rupert. He apparently didn't think about Luce and I didn't think about Anaïs.

The affair that started that night went on for some time, but only when Anaïs was absent from Rupert's bed. Luce raised no objection to my interludes with Rupert, perhaps because in that era a lesbian relationship was not necessarily to be taken seriously when a man entered the picture. Was this turn of events outrageous? Yes. Should it have happened? No, but it did. I reveled in the attentions of this gorgeous man and just assumed that Luce would be there when I got home. And she was.

With fitting irony, Anaïs decided at one point that I should meet her other husband, Hugo, when we happened to be in Acapulco at the same time. The three of us had a lovely dinner under the stars. I was almost breathless with the intrigue of it—what I knew about Anaïs and what she didn't know about me.

Forty-three years later, in 1995, Deidre Bair published her massive 654-page biography of Anaïs Nin. I spent many hours talking to Deidre about Anaïs, but I ended up with one line in the book: "So she kept on going to Rupert and the life she despised, only to discover something she had always feared: that Rupert was in the midst of a long affair with her friend Betty Berzon." How titillating to be forever recorded as the "other woman" in the life of so quintessential an "other woman" as Anaïs Nin. I would much rather have been represented by another story I had told Deidre Bair.

One day I got a phone call from a very reputable book dealer I knew. He said he had for sale some typewritten erotica by Anaïs Nin. He knew that I handled her books, and he thought I might know of a potential buyer. Discretion was the order of the day because selling typewritten pornography at that time was illegal. I immediately called Anaïs to tell her about it.

"Oh my god," she said. "Those pages were never to be made public. I can't believe this."

She told me the story of the group of impoverished young New York writers who had signed up to write anonymous, made-to-order erotica for a dollar a page. Some of these writers had since become quite famous. The intermediary, through whom the arrangement was made, swore not to reveal to the writers who the client was and not to reveal to the client the identity of the writers. These pages were never to be seen by anyone but the principal parties.

Anaïs was disturbed to learn that this pornography was not only on the market but that her name appeared as the author. "I must see these pages," she said almost hysterically.

"Well, I don't think he'll let them out of his store."

"Then I'll go there."

"Don't be ridiculous, Anaïs. He'll recognize you and refuse to even admit he has these illegal manuscripts."

"I'll go in disguise!"

I rolled my eyes. It would have to be one hell of a disguise to hide that distinctive face. She assured me it would work. Unconvinced but lacking the will to fight her, I took a deep breath and called the dealer to tell him I had a potential buyer for his pornography.

Anaïs arrived at my bookstore dressed for an early horror flick—long black coat and a hat with a veil so thick it totally obscured her face. I told her that she must under no circumstances speak. She had made audio recordings of much of her writing and her voice was as distinctive as her face. She agreed to remain silent.

When we arrived at the bookshop, I introduced Anaïs as Mrs. Smith. The dealer led us up a flight of stairs to a balcony at the back of the store. He unlocked a cabinet and spread the pages of the manuscript on a table before us. Anaïs lifted her veil ever so slightly and peered at the pages. Slowly she turned them, then suddenly she groaned and began to moan. I gave the dealer a knowing look. He looked a little embarrassed and took his leave. As soon as he was gone Anaïs pushed the veil off her face and began poring over the pages.

"Oh, god, this is it. I never wanted to see these pages again. I'm sick. That's enough. Let's get out of here."

She replaced her veil and started down the stairs. Startled, I followed as she hurried toward the front door. The dealer looked puzzled. I shrugged my shoulders and told him I would call him as I scurried to keep up with the fleeing Anaïs. In the car I asked if she was okay.

"I don't know whether to laugh or cry," she said, tearing off her hat. "How naive we were to think we would be protected. I hated being ordered to reduce the power and magic of sex to mere mechanics. I hated what I was doing and now it's out there with my name on it."

"Well, Mrs. Smith, I guess there's nothing you can do about it now."

To illustrate how evolving mores bring about change, in 1977 I picked up a copy of *Delta of Venus: Erotica by Anaïs Nin.* It was those same pages, no longer sold illicitly under the counter, but published by Harcourt Brace Jovanovich, and a book club selection.

My friendship with Anaïs continued through the postbookstore days when I experienced a painful reorganization of my life. She was helpful to me in those first weeks and months. Her own career flourished, and with the publication of her diaries in 1966, she became a commercial success. By then Rupert was no longer a forest ranger but was teaching science in the Los Angeles public schools. They lived in a lovely glass house overlooking Silver Lake, designed by Rupert's stepbrother, architect Eric Wright. Somewhere along the way, in the chaos my life would become, Anaïs and I lost touch. One evening at a dinner party in the 1970s, I was seated next to my old friend James Leo Herlihy. Jamie was as close to Anaïs Nin as anyone, except Rupert. She called Jamie her "writing twin." He told me that Anaïs

70

was dying and he was spending most of his time sitting with her. He had just returned from a quick flight to Japan to obtain a drug not sold in this county that they hoped would prolong her life a bit. It did, but not for long. Anaïs Nin died in that lovely glass house on the hill overlooking Silver Lake, January 14, 1977, just before her seventy-fourth birthday.

For all the success I believed I was having, by mid-1951 I was beginning to feel the strain of running a business and keeping up with the social whirl that had evolved out of the back of the bookstore scene. I was not only working twelve-hour days, but going out to eat and drink afterward, often until 2 A.M. I was only vaguely aware that I was beginning to fray around the edges.

Financial problems were also beginning to worry me. No one had told me not to live off my capital, so I went merrily along spending down my assets before the business had grown enough for profits to offset expenses. The dwindling balance in my checkbook told me that I was headed for trouble.

I was saved by the arrival of Lila's friend, Brook, a deus ex machina if ever there was one. He was enthralled with the bookstore, he had been thinking of moving to Los Angeles, and, yes, he would love to become my partner. Most important, he had family money to invest. I was ecstatic, promising to teach him all about the book business. He was delighted to have found this new challenge and to be with his friends again.

By this time, Luce and I were living in a charming garden apartment, two bedrooms upstairs and a two-story living room. Close by our front door a little stream meandered through the garden, goldfish darting in and out among the rocks. It was very peaceful there on Fuller Avenue.

Just before Brook's move to Los Angeles, as if by a miracle, the apartment next to ours came up for rent. It was perfect for Brook and for us because there was a secret passage through two upstairs closets that connected our apartments, which meant that Brook's poodle and Luce's cocker spaniel, already friends, could cavort from one apartment to the other.

Brook's presence in the bookstore helped for a while, but soon the pace of my life began catching up with me again. The merry-go-round was going too fast. Too many people, not enough sleep, too many problems, not enough time. I had little energy left for Luce, which she resented, and I resented her just hanging out in the back of the store not working. The more tension grew between us, the more time I put into the business. Our relationship was unraveling and neither of us had any idea what to do about it. We didn't know how to talk about problems, so we just each reverted to our own tried-and-true escape routes: I worked, she started an affair.

I tried to ignore what I knew was happening and concentrated on keeping up with the crowd, hoping that parties, drinking, and dancing would drown out the pain. Everything felt speeded up, more intense. The music got louder, images blurred into one another, everyone seemed to be screaming to be heard.

Then Luce came to me and said, "I'm leaving," and all motion stopped. I came home one night to find Luce's things gone, the dog gone, the secret passage closed off. I was devastated. All I could feel was confusion and excruciating pain.

I stopped going to the bookstore. I walked. I drove. I wandered. I went from nowhere to nowhere. I couldn't separate myself from the agony. I went over a thousand scenarios in my head: she left me because I was unlovable, because I was a terrible lover, because I didn't know how to be a lesbian, because I didn't give her enough money. What I didn't think about was that she left me because I put her down, ignored, rejected, and invalidated her.

Brook soon began to lose patience with me. He was floundering in the store because he didn't know the book business, but I didn't care about that. I didn't care about anything. I could connect only with the sinking feeling, the constant feeling that I was sinking inside.

Days went by. I stayed in bed. I stopped eating. I didn't answer the phone. I lost touch with everyone. I became so cut off that I felt more and more detached and frightened, but the fear felt good in an odd way, better than the emptiness. Connecting with the fear was like venturing onto a path leading back to reality. I didn't know what I was afraid of, but it seemed to be something outside myself, and that is exactly what I needed to do, get outside myself. I had to find someone who would understand. I thought I knew who that could be, though I didn't exactly know why. I went to see Lila.

If Lila felt any satisfaction at my now being in the position I had put her in, she didn't show it. Instead, she told me she thought I was going through a serious depression and I needed to get help. I remember staring at her, wondering what she meant by "help."

I told Lila that I was thinking of killing myself, seemingly the only way to get rid of the pain, and that I thought I might need help to accomplish that. She said she understood how I felt, but that wasn't what she meant by "help."

"Sit right there," she said. "I'm going to make a phone call. I'll be right back."

When Lila returned, she sat next to me and spoke very gently. "I've talked to a doctor friend who told me about a place you can go for a while until you feel better. They'll take care of you and help you get through this depression. My friend can make the arrangements."

Childlike, I questioned her, "Do you think I should do it?"

"Yes," she said, "I think you should do it, and I'll take you there now, if you want me to."

7

As we drove up the long, winding driveway of Resthaven I felt doubt that I should be doing this, then comfort at the thought of being taken care of, then doubt again. Lila came with me into the building, where we were asked to wait in the lobby. Soon we were approached by a rather stiff-looking young woman cradling a clipboard in her arm. She looked from one of us to the other. Through my fog I felt amused at what I realized was happening. "I'm the patient," I said.

The clipboard lady asked a lot of questions. What I couldn't answer, Lila did, identifying herself as a close friend. When the questioning was over, the social worker, as I later learned she was, introduced us to Resthaven. It was an open psychiatric hospital with a closed staff. That meant one could only be treated by a doctor already on staff. I would be assigned to one of the doctors. The open hospital meant no locked doors, but the rule was strict—once a patient took "French leave," there was no coming back. Because Resthaven was partially supported by county money, charges were based on ability to pay. That would be discussed later.

I was still not really sure that I wanted to be a patient in a psychiatric hospital, but I knew I was in trouble and I did feel a glimmer of hope at the possibility of feeling better.

Resthaven lived up to its name. I felt safe there. I liked it. It didn't smell like a hospital or have any of the sounds of a hospital. It was more like a hotel, quiet and a little mysterious. My tiny private room became my world. I spent a lot of time pacing, which gave me the illusion of being in control of myself, something I needed to feel after days of fearing that I would never be in control of my life again.

I left my room for meals and "chats" with the social worker. The chats didn't feel productive to me because I hadn't yet told her my "secret." On the fourth day, at the end of the interview, she asked if there was anything else I wanted to tell her. I got up and went to the door. "I am a homosexual," I blurted out, and quickly left the room.

The next day I felt nervous going for my chat. I had summoned up thoughts of the social worker shaking her head in shock at my revelation as soon as the door had closed. On entering the room this day I searched her face for signs of disgust. There were none. She was her same unresponsive self.

By the end of the second week I still had not been assigned to a doctor, but it didn't matter. I was feeling better, on vacation from the world, away from the pressures of business and the social whirl, moving through my days in slow motion, thinking of Luce most of the time. I was becalmed, sleeping, eating, writing poetry, and waiting. I began to believe in the possibility that someday I could be all right again.

I was puzzled about why I was never assigned to a doctor. Then, the issue became moot. I was summoned to the infirmary to have a checkup. When the examination was over I was told to sit in the waiting room. I dutifully sat, though I wasn't sure what I was waiting for. Soon a woman, who I assumed to be another patient, came in and sat next to me. She tried to make conversation, but I wasn't really interested. Then she made what seemed a last ditch effort to engage me. "You know why you had that physical, don't you?"

"No," I answered, "I don't know."

She stood and moved to the window. "Come here." Reluctantly, I went. She pointed across the courtyard. "You see that line of people out there, waiting to go into that building?"

"Yes."

"They are waiting to get their electroshock treatments."

"Their what?"

"Shock treatments. They strap you to a bed and zap your brain with electricity. It's a little like getting electrocuted."

"Why do they do that?" I asked, horrified.

"It's supposed to cure your depression. What you don't see is these same people being carried out the other side after they're zapped."

"Where are they carried to?"

She said they were carried back to their rooms to regain consciousness. My eyes were riveted on the line across the courtyard. Did the Jews at Auschwitz stand in line so passively waiting for the ovens? I knew what she was about to say before she said it.

"You're next. They always give you a physical before they zap."

"But I haven't even seen a psychiatrist yet."

"You will very soon now."

Shuddering, I looked back at the line of people. I had to get out of this place! I left the infirmary and walked back to my room, slowly, not wanting to attract any attention to myself. In the room I pulled on a sweater and carefully put two items into my shirt pocket, my driver's license and a tiny book I'd received as a Christmas gift—a lecture on James Joyce by Italo Svevo, translated into English by Joyce's brother, Stanislaus. I had identification and something to read. I walked to the front hall of the building and waited until the entryway was empty. Then I opened the door and walked out of Resthaven. I felt immediately relieved.

I had no destination in mind. Resthaven was near downtown Los Angeles, and I descended the hilly street in that direction. I only knew that I had to get away, to escape the electrocutioners. After walking half an hour, I saw the clock tower of Union Station rising above the red-tiled roof of the terminal. That became my destination.

I felt very calm as I entered the train station. The roar of conversation in the high-ceilinged room was a backdrop to the bulleted announcements on the public address system of arrivals and departures. Train travel at that time was still the main way people got around in this country and the terminal was buzzing.

I didn't think about what I was going to do, I just did it. I went toward the departure gates behind which the trains were backed up, waiting to be boarded. When the ticket taker was momentarily distracted, I scurried past, unnoticed. I walked along the platform beside one of the trains until I got to a middle car, then I grabbed a handrail and swung myself up the steps and into the vestibule. Pulling open the heavy metal door, I let myself into the car.

Once inside, I flashed back to train trips with my mother, going back and forth between St. Louis and Tucson. The war was still on then and every car was jammed with servicemen standing in the aisles for part of the journey, trading off with their buddies who had seats. Here it was again, the cloying odor of too many bodies in one place, the acrid smell of cigarette smoke that everybody took for granted as a part of the air they breathed.

I plopped wearily into a seat. Soon the train lurched forward and began moving. We were about ten minutes out of Union Station when the conductor came through collecting tickets. I made a dash for the ladies room. I sat in front of the mirror, staring at my face but not really seeing myself. I was lost in reverie when the woman came in and sat down. She carefully pulled on the hatpin to remove her hat, tossing her hair free. I watched in silence. Seeing that I was watching her, she smiled. I smiled back.

"I barely made this train," she said sighing. "I was at work when I got the call that my daughter has to have an operation tomorrow. I just ran out the door. I packed so fast I'm not even sure what's in that suitcase."

I watched her combing her hair, checking her makeup. Without looking at me she asked, "Where are you going, dear?"

"I don't know. Where is this train going?"

The hand with the comb paused in midair. She turned to look at me. "You don't know where the train is going? Why are you on it?"

The thought of shocking this woman sent a little curl of excitement up my back. "Well, I just escaped from a sanitarium and I have to go somewhere. Where *is* this train going?"

The woman froze for a moment, then she hastily gathered up her things. At the door she gave me a long look, then disappeared. Several minutes later there was a knock at the door, and the conductor stuck his head in. "Tickets?" I dropped my head to the counter. Pointing back toward the car I groaned, "My husband has it."

"Okay, hope you feel better."

I took my little book out and began to read. About five minutes later, the door opened again. The conductor stood in the doorway. I could see the woman in the hat just behind him. The conductor said in a stern voice, "Would you step out here, miss?" As I stepped into the corridor, the woman nodded to the conductor and scurried away. The conductor said, "Come with me." I followed him to a seat at the back of the car.

"Okay, now, who are you?"

I told him my name.

"Do you have a ticket for this train?"

"No."

"Then why are you on this train?"

I told him what I'd told the woman in the hat.

"I see. I'm going to have to put you off at the next stop. Sit right here and don't move. You won't move will you?"

"No sir."

Whatever illusion of control over my fate that I'd managed so far to sustain was gone again. When the conductor reappeared he said, "We'll be stopping in a few minutes in Saugus. There will be someone to meet you there." I'd never heard of Saugus. Who could possibly be there to meet me?

The train jerked to a stop and the conductor took me by the arm and walked me onto the platform. Two uniformed deputy sheriffs were waiting.

A hushed conversation ensued between the deputies and the conductor. I heard words like "crazy" and "escaped." The deputies were shaking their heads and I heard "no jurisdiction." With that, the deputies walked away, leaving the conductor muttering something I couldn't quite hear.

The next thing I knew I was being shoved into the waiting room of the train station, a one-story yellow clapboard building with windows all around. "Sit down in there and don't move!" the conductor angrily commanded. He went away and came back with the ticket clerk. "You have to call someone to come and pick you up."

"I don't know anyone to call."

"Fine," the conductor said, and he stormed out of the station leaving me alone with the clerk.

"Are you certain you don't know who to call? I could do that for you," the clerk said.

I shook my head.

"Well, I'm sorry, but I have to lock you in here. We'll use the waiting room on the other side of the station. If you want anything, just tap on the ticket window over there. Uh, it's gonna be all right, honey, I'm sure," he said nervously. "Just stay calm."

The door clicked shut behind him, locking me in. I wondered what kind of a threat he thought I was. I didn't think I looked menacing, but I guess you never can tell with crazy people.

I looked around my little prison, row upon row of rounded yellow wooden benches. The wrap-around windows afforded a view of the railroad yard and some ramshackle houses beyond. It was quiet, the kind of stillness you feel just before something momentous happens.

I opened my tiny book and stretched out on one of the benches. I had been reading for several minutes when I heard a commotion outside, voices and laughter. I went to the window. Three boys were standing just outside the waiting room. They looked to be ten or eleven. When they saw me, they sprang into action. One picked up a handful of gravel from the ground and heaved it at the window. The other two began to jump and shout. At first, I couldn't make out what they were shouting. Then I understood. All three were now throwing gravel at the window and chanting in sing-song voices.

"CRAZY LADY! CRAZY LADY! CRAZY LADY!"

I closed my eyes and put my hands over my ears, but I could still hear them. How did they know? Who told them?

"CRAZY LADY! CRAZY LADY! CRAZY LADY!"

My head was reeling. Was this my Greek chorus come to pronounce my fate? The voices grew more shrill. The gravel pinged against the window in steady accompaniment to the chanting. I couldn't stand it, but I couldn't shut them out. I had to make it stop. I banged on the ticket window. It flew open and the clerk appeared.

"What's happening?" he asked.

"Make them stop! Please make them stop!"

The clerk leaned out of the ticket window far enough to see the boys. "Aw, they're just a bunch of kids. I told them to stay away from this side of the building."

He'd probably told them why too. The clerk shut the window and went outside to shoo the boys away. It was quiet again, but I could still hear the chorus in my head.

"CRAZY LADY! CRAZY LADY! CRAZY LADY!"

What was I doing here? Fragments of the day came back to me. The lineup that I'd seen outside the window at Resthaven. My escape. Boarding the train. The woman in the hat. The conductor. Being thrown off the train, locked in the station. I felt disoriented, confused. I looked around the bleak waiting room and began to sense the sinking feeling again. I was alone, abandoned, no one to turn to, the sadness taking over.

I sat staring into space, dulled to the sounds of trains moving in the yards, of voices, of feet crunching on the gravel outside, bits and pieces of meaning that came and went in my head, barely registering at the edges of my awareness. And then, suddenly, I was shaking myself awake. As mysteriously as my decisions had come to me all day, I knew what I had to do. I tapped on the ticket window. The clerk appeared.

"I've thought of someone to call."

Lila arrived about two hours later.

It's 1994. Lila and I are having lunch at the Union Square Cafe in New York City.

"Do you remember the trip from Saugus back to Resthaven?" she asks.

"No, I don't. Why? What happened?"

Lila laughs. "You decided to commit suicide by jumping out of the car while we were on the highway. You kept opening the door. I had to drive with one hand and hold onto you with the other."

"Oh my god! How terrible for you! I have absolutely no memory of that."

"Just as well," Lila says.

I look at this person who had clearly saved my life, who had become a loyal friend to me in return for my betrayal of her. "I'm sorry about the wild ride. I'm sorry about Luce," I say.

"Please. No need to be sorry about either one. It was several lifetimes ago."

Having rescued myself from Resthaven and the zappers, I next began outpatient therapy at the Los Angeles Psychiatric Service, fifty cents per session, take what you get by way of a therapist. My first draw was with a young French psychiatrist, new to this country and to the English language. I told him my situation, and he listened carefully, then asked a question.

"Do you like lesbians?"

I didn't know how to answer that. "I do and I don't," I said.

"When you are with lesbians, do you lick them?"

I was horrified. "I think I'll leave now," I said on my way out the door.

Determined to get help, I requested another therapist and was assigned to a young psychiatrist just out of his residency. His name was Fred Feldman. I saw him for a brief time at LAPS, then in his new office in Beverly Hills. When he moved I told him I couldn't afford him anymore, but he insisted that I continue to see him anyway. "You'll be my annuity," he said. I did see him for the next four years. He didn't charge me. I do not believe I would be alive today if it were not for Fred Feldman.

I saw Dr. Feldman weekly, and I moved from the apartment on Fuller to a tiny two-room studio in West Hollywood. New surroundings helped me adjust to the reality of no longer being with Luce. I was on my own again, a circumstance about which I had mixed feelings—sadness at the loss of my relationship but also relief that I no longer had to be concerned about Luce needing my attention, Luce not working, or Luce using my shop as a social base. I didn't have to be concerned about Luce at all, though I still thought about her more than I wanted to.

I returned to the bookstore to try to mend fences with Brook and salvage what I could of the business. The fence mending didn't go well. Brook came to the store less and less, glad (I'm sure) to extricate himself from my problems. Much of my focus then was on fighting depression. There was no help to find in the pharmacy, antidepressants hadn't been invented yet. Instead,

I was staying out of the bars and away from the partying crowd. I felt breakable, too fragile to subject myself to anything that might trigger depression.

It is July 4, 1951, and I am having a terrible dream. Luce is running away from me, I am chasing her, begging her to stop. Sometimes I get close enough to touch her. I reach out, but she slips away. Looking over her shoulder, she laughs at me, taunting, mocking, her face going from beautiful to grotesque. I scream at her, "Please, please, stop!" She turns and mouths the words, "I love you." Then she disappears into thin air. I run faster, but she is nowhere to be seen. I am desperate to find her. I awaken in an agitated state.

I have no plans for this holiday. I decide to go to the bookstore to do some work, but when I get there I am unable to concentrate. I can only look blankly at the papers on my desk. My mind slips back to the dream, and I feel the agitation all over again. Why is Luce so elusive? Why won't she let me catch her, touch her, be with her? I close my eyes and give myself over to the feelings, the despair, but wait, I'm not in the dream now. I know where Luce is. I can call her. I reach for the phone and dial the number. It rings over and over. No answer.

Maybe I dialed wrong. Try again. It rings six, seven, ten times. I can feel the anger building inside. Why is she doing this to me? I can't stand being so helpless. It infuriates me. Why does she have such power over me? I hate her. I want to crush her, destroy her.

I hurl the phone against the wall. It bounces, rings, and lies still. With the full force of my anger, I sweep my arm across the desk, crashing everything to the floor. I feel the fury now. I see the books, the books that kept me from Luce, that demanded so much of me. I begin pulling the books from the shelves, faster and faster until the floor is covered with them, and when the shelves are empty, I pull the bookcases down on top of the piles of books.

I pick my way through the rubble to the back of the store where the parties were that I never had time to attend. I smack the coffee cups and glasses out of the cabinets and onto to the floor. The backs of my hands are raw and bloody. I upend tables and chairs, flailing wildly at the debris, nothing whole, nothing upright. I grab a large piece of butcher paper and scrawl across it in big, crazy letters: "CLOSED FOREVER!" and shove it into the front window of the shop, dropping the metal blinds until they fall crooked, hanging in a drunken slant behind the window. I sink into the piles of books on the floor, the books I had so dearly loved, and I cry, wracking sobs. I know I will never be all right again now. I have just destroyed my work and my life.

I've no idea how much time passed before I came to and saw the chaos around me. What happened? Who did this? My brain was foggy as I looked around the wrecked bookstore. The truth slowly came into focus. I felt horribly ashamed and frightened. I needed to get help.

When Dr. Feldman came on the line I told him what I had done. He asked questions, then he said he was going to tell me exactly what to do, that I should listen carefully and stop him if I didn't understand anything. Did I think I could drive? Yes, I thought so. I was to drive to a certain pharmacy in Hollywood where they would have a pill for me to take immediately. I should wait half an hour then drive to the Westerly Sanitarium, where they would be expecting me. He slowly explained the directions.

"Do you think you can do that?"

"Yes, but what am I doing?"

"You're admitting yourself to a hospital until you get through this period of agitation. I will see you there later this afternoon. Don't worry. I'll arrange everything. Just go. If you get confused on the way, stop and call me again."

As I look back on these events now, I am astonished that I was actually sent to a pharmacy to take a pill (a barbiturate, no tranquilizers yet), told to drive a car, find my way to a hospital, and admit myself as a patient. Although I indeed followed these instructions, it all seems as unbelievable to me now as my rampage in the bookstore itself.

The Westerly Sanitarium was a sprawling property near Santa Monica. Well-tended grounds and whitewashed buildings presented a picture of order and tranquility. I rang the bell at the front entrance. The nurse was expecting me as I'd been told, and she admitted me, smiling and putting her arm around me. When I heard the heavy metal door slam shut and click behind me, clearly locking, I knew this was going to be serious business.

Exhausted, I slept as soon as I hit my room. When I awoke a few hours later my eyes went to the window and the bars covering it. A chill went through me. What had I gotten myself into here? Then I saw my hands. Little rivulets of congealed blood crisscrossed the back of each hand in neat, almost orderly, patterns. I was studying my hands as the door opened and a nurse entered. She was starched white and gratingly cheerful. "And are we feeling better?" she chirped.

I didn't answer.

The nurse got a washcloth from the sink and began washing the blood off my hands. I watched in silence as she applied lotion to the raw skin. I didn't like having my wounds cleaned. They seemed like wounds of dishonor that I should keep to remind me of my destructive behavior. I was horrified to think of what I had done. I had to understand it. Who or what was I trying to kill?

My reverie was interrupted by the entrance of Dr. Feldman. He listened to my story, then he said he was sorry that I'd thought I needed to see Luce, that in the future I should not see or try to contact Luce again, that any feelings or dreams I had about her I should tell him. He also suggested that it might be time to think about giving up the bookstore and concentrating on getting well. It was a relief to hear him say that, and I felt a burden lift.

Dr. Feldman suggested I stay at the Westerly for a few weeks. He'd called my father, who said he would pay for it. I knew, of course, my father would renege on the payment and he did. He didn't pay and he didn't visit, but his promise bought me the few weeks rest and treatment I needed.

My first week at the Westerly I was restricted to the locked ward. Meals on a tray. No activities. A lot of time to calm down and think. I had no decisions to make. What I could and could not do was controlled by other people, which gave me comfort. I lived in a circumscribed space, physically and mentally, where I was safe from myself.

After a few days I began to look around at the other patients on the ward. One in particular fascinated me, a beautiful young girl, Melinda, who floated silently around the halls, always in motion going nowhere. There was something about Melinda that was intriguing. Though I realized that this sixteen-year-old girl was probably quite crazy, the ability to detach from reality so effectively had a certain attraction. I tried to talk to Melinda, but she looked right through me as though I didn't exist. Then came the day when she decided to murder me. I was sitting in the day room reading a magazine.

"I'm going to have to kill you," Melinda said. She was standing over me, having floated into the room without my noticing. Looking into her face I did not feel frightened. She seemed too ethereal to be taken seriously.

"Why do you have to kill me?" I asked.

"Because you are disturbing me," Melinda said in a flat voice.

"I'm sorry. I wanted to get to know you. I didn't mean to bother you."

"Nobody can know me," Melinda said angrily. "That's why I have to kill you."

At that point Melinda brought the weapon of death from behind her back. It was a handful of daffodils that she threw at me with all her might. I clutched at my abdomen, groaned, and pitched forward to the floor. Melinda began to laugh wildly. "You see! You see! Nobody can know me!" And giving my body a kick, she ran out the door.

Having survived Melinda's attack, I stayed on the floor awhile, thinking. This crazy child had lost the ability to know fantasy from reality. Maybe that is what happened to me in the bookstore. Was I so overwhelmed by the fantasy of striking out at Luce that I lost touch with the reality of what I was actually destroying? But that was a temporary lapse. Now I knew all too well what I did, and I was beginning to see that it wasn't Luce that I needed to get rid of as much as it was the sexual attraction that drew me to her. Suddenly, it seemed clear that being a homosexual was at the root of all my problems.

In the days to come I spent many sessions with Dr. Feldman talking about my fear that homosexuality would continue to ruin my life. He said he wasn't at all sure that I really was homosexual, but I certainly didn't have to be. We would work on it together. I felt renewed hope that I could be a normal person. In my next two weeks at the Westerly I was granted more freedom, meals in the dining room, occupational therapy, volleyball, shuffleboard. I was beginning to feel sociable again, relating to other patients, even joining in their little joke about our regimented existence at the hospital. Staff members escorted patient groups from one activity to the next. We weren't required to march in lockstep, but when the staff turned away we all feigned a goose step and "heiled" our attendant. It was interesting that these groups of eight or ten, in varying stages of impairment and recovery, could collaborate to make a joke.

After three weeks of a variety of therapies, I felt stitched back together. The seams were still showing, but I had a program with Dr. Feldman that made me optimistic about the future. I felt ready to face the world again, and in early August, I was discharged.

For what was left of the summer, I did what was necessary to close the bookstore. Brook finally gave up on getting his money back from me. He did go on to become a prominent university librarian, so I had helped him on his way in that regard, but he never again had anything much to say to me.

I rarely saw my own family during this period. My mother was preoccupied with survival as a single parent. My father was busy with his marriage to Mrs. Green, by then Mrs. Berzon Number Two, in later years to be succeeded by the third, fourth, fifth, and sixth Mrs. Berzons. Mrs. Green did not seem especially perturbed about the loss of the bookstore. She was a businesswoman and took such things in stride.

I was doing pretty well, thinking of returning to finish my undergraduate work and going on to library school. The one thing I felt most confident about was that I wasn't ever going to be homosexual again. I was finished with that part of my life.

And then, one day, Luce called me.

I was surprised. She said she'd heard I was feeling better and maybe we could get together, have dinner or something. She said she missed me and hoped we could be friends. Dr. Feldman's warning rang in my ears. I told myself that seeing Luce was not a good idea, that it was dangerous for me to be involved with her, that her leaving had turned my life inside out. I told myself all that, and then I said, "Sure, let's get together."

We met for dinner. As soon as I saw her all the old feelings came back. I was excited to be with her. I was embarrassed that I'd handled the relationship so badly. We talked about what had happened to each of us, only I edited out the more dramatic details of my recent life. When dinner was over I suggested we go back to my place, and she readily agreed. We were awkward with each other at first, but after a few glasses of wine we gradually relaxed. She told me that she had been afraid to contact me, but she was glad now that she had. I was overwhelmed by desire to feel her close to me, to have my body against hers again. Hesitantly, I took her hand and led her into the bedroom. She followed willingly.

On the bed I held tightly to her, as though to make up in minutes for what I'd been missing for months. It was as if we were discovering each other all over again. This was the person who had brought me to life in such an important way. I could feel myself opening to her with all the same excitement that I'd felt our first time together. I forgot everything but the ecstasy of being with her. I was whole again. Luce was back.

Then, suddenly, she sat up. She looked at her watch.

"Well, I have to be going now," she said.

I didn't understand what I was hearing. She couldn't mean she was leaving.

"Maybe we can have dinner again sometime soon," she said.

I felt confused, then frightened. I could feel the anger coming. She was leaving again. It didn't occur to me to ask why. My head felt like it was exploding. I jumped off the bed and screamed at her.

"All right, go! Just go! Get out right now!"

She stammered, "Well, I didn't mean to . . . I mean . . . please don't get angry."

But I was beyond anger, I was reeling.

"Just go! Just get out!"

She gathered her things and went to the door, where she paused, looking at me with the same puzzled frown I had seen so many times. Then she turned and walked through the door. That was the last time I ever saw Luce.

At first, I just stood in the middle of the room staring at the door. I told myself that I must not lose control, but even as the thought formed I could feel the anger engulfing me. I rammed my fists against the door, pounding until my hands were too sore to continue. I ranged around the room looking for something to throw. No, I will not destroy things this time. What I really wanted to destroy was whatever it was inside me that made me so vulnerable to this woman, to my need for her, the desire she aroused in me. I hated it. I hated her. I hated myself.

I sat on the floor, rocking back and forth. *Hold on. Don't let go.* I cradled myself and rocked, a mother holding a child. I was the mother and the child. All I could think of was how much I hurt. I wanted the pain to go away. Then, something clicked. I stood up and went into the bathroom, took a razor blade out of the medicine chest. I began to feel a strange calm. In the bedroom, I sat down and slowly, methodically drew the razor blade across the back of my hand. I cut again and again until my hands were raked and bloody. Those little rivulets of blood were back, crisscrossing in orderly patterns, the familiar wounds of the bookstore. Then I turned my hand over and began slicing at the veins in my wrist.

At first I didn't cut deeply and only tiny bubbles of blood appeared. Then I cut harder and the blood began to flow in a steady stream down my upraised arm, spreading across my lap and onto the bed. I watched as the deepening red stain grew larger. I cut again, intent now only on this task. I felt dizzy. The walls of my tiny bedroom began to move. I had to finish what I was doing before the walls crashed in on me. Hurriedly, I sliced at my wrist, hardly able to see what I was doing through my tears.

Suddenly exhausted, I fell back against the pillows. I was very tired, too tired to do anymore. I wanted to sleep, but I felt afraid to sleep. Then I realized with a start that if I slept I was going to die. Inside me a tiny voice began to protest. I didn't want to die. I just wanted to be rid of the pain. I sat up and grabbed my arm. Holding on to the wall, I walked unsteadily into the bathroom and wrapped a towel tightly around my wrist. Back in the bedroom, I dialed Dr. Feldman's number and got his answering service.

"I have to talk to Dr. Feldman," I said. "I've just cut my wrist and I'm bleeding badly."

The woman on the other end replied in a calm voice. "Tell me your name and where you are calling from."

I felt annoyed, but I answered her questions. "I need to talk to him now."

"Stay on the line. I'll call him right away."

I was losing focus. I wanted to sleep. It seemed forever until Dr. Feldman came on the line. I told him what I had done. His tone was steady, but I also heard the note of alarm in his voice. He said, "I'm sending an ambulance. Stay where you are. What's your address?"

I told him. "Please hurry," I pleaded.

I lay back on the bed. The walls were moving again. I closed my eyes, telling myself to hang on. Within minutes I heard the siren. I rose with difficulty and moved toward the front door, walking as in a dream. I opened the door and leaned against it. My vision was clouding, I tried to concentrate on the two white-clad figures hurrying toward me, but they began to blur, then everything blurred and went dark.

There are moments forever etched in memory, indelible imprints. I will never forget waking up in that hospital bed, seeing the leather restraints on my ankles, my bandaged wrists tethered to the bed rails. I couldn't move. I was helpless, trapped.

I wondered where I was. The walls were a soft blue, a metal chair in the corner. The single window was barred. I glanced at the table beside the bed, where a rack held two towels. I strained to see the printing stamped on them: "The Westerly." I was back. What a disappointment I was to myself. What a disappointment I must be to Dr. Feldman. How could I have been so weak, so foolish as to see Luce again? I had no willpower, no sense. I belonged in a hospital restrained like this. I couldn't be trusted. I'd conned myself, believing like a naive child that I could see Luce and that it would be all right. The door opened and a nurse came in.

"Well, glad you're awake. How are you feeling?"

There was none of the resistance I had felt my first time at the Westerly. "I feel tired and my hands hurt. Do I have to be trussed up like this?"

"Just until the doctor tells us the restraints can come off."

Dr. Feldman arrived shortly after that and the restraints were removed. "Are you mad at me?" I asked like a contrite child.

"No, I'm just glad you rescued yourself." His face softened and he put his hand on my arm. "I just want you to be all right," he said.

I felt more strongly than ever before that he really cared about me. I vowed not to disappoint him, or myself, again. This was going to be the turning point. I told him he could trust me now, and I must have convinced him because the restraints came off for good.

In the next few weeks my sessions with Dr. Feldman were very productive. I was eager to be the good patient, to please him, to get well. Once again he reassured me that I did not have to be homosexual and I assured him that I would work hard not to be. Soon I was feeling stable again and strong enough to join the other residents in the dining room and at activities. My hands were healed sufficiently for the bandages to be removed. They were not a pretty sight; I usually kept them in my pockets or behind my back, and I no longer felt intrigued by my wounds. I just wanted them to heal and be over with.

I was much more sociable with the other patients this time around. I found I was particularly interested in their stories. Why were they in the hospital? What had happened in their lives to bring them to this point? How did they feel now? What did they think was going to happen to them? No one seemed to mind these discussions; in fact, I think they liked the attention. I didn't know why I was drawn to talk to these people so candidly, but doing so fascinated me.

I was especially curious about one patient in particular. Dorothy Comingore was an actress who had risen to stardom almost overnight when she played Orson Welles's wife in the film *Citizen Kane*. She was as bright as she was beautiful, but her life had become a nightmare after she appeared as an "unfriendly witness" before the House Un-American Activities Committee. Divorce and a bitter custody battle were further complicated by excessive drinking.

Dorothy and I talked for long hours about how one could maintain a sense of equilibrium while being battered by enemies from within and without. I felt as if she and I had in common an internal conflict about reconcil-

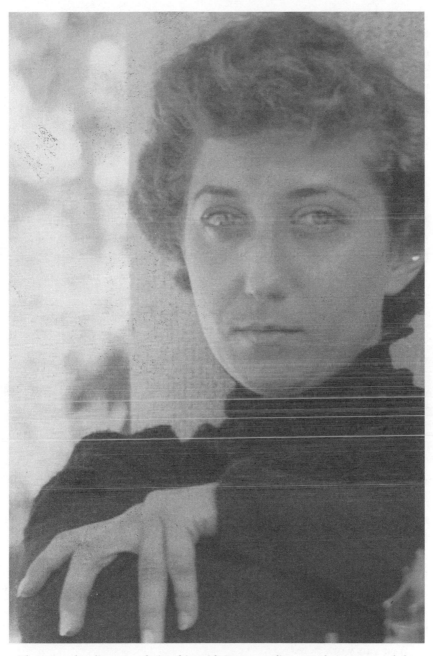

The pain of ending my relationship with Luce, my distress at being gay, and the pressure of working fourteen-hour days became too much. I unraveled and spent a year in and out of psychiatric hospitals.

ing our identities. Because of the intensity of our exchanges and our conviction that we helped one another, Dorothy was instrumental in the extraordinary turn my life was about to take.

It was just after Christmas and I was ready to be discharged. Don Babbidge, the administrative director of the Westerly, asked me to go for a walk. Don, in his late thirties, was a lanky redhead with a face full of freckles. A hands-on administrator, he took meals with the patients, participated in recreational activities, and walked the wards every day. All the patients were on a first-name basis with him.

Don and I strolled around the grounds talking about the hospital and its programs. I was bracing to be told that my insurance wasn't going to cover any of my hospitalization or that my father had declined to pay his part of the bill, but neither topic seemed to be on the agenda. Don finally came to the point.

"What are you going to do when you leave here?"

"I'm planning to go to library school."

"Have you ever thought of becoming a psychologist?"

"A *what?*"

"A psychologist, working with people."

"No," I laughed. "I've never had such a thought. My whole life has been about books. And anyway, what kind of a psychologist would I make having been a patient in a place like this?"

"An especially good one, I think."

"Are you serious?"

"Very serious."

"Hey, what is this all about? Why would you think of *me* as a psychologist?"

"Because I've heard you talking to some of the patients. You get them to open up to you. They like talking to you. Several people have told me that. I think you might have a talent for working with people."

I stopped and stared at Don. I was astonished. I didn't know what to say. He went on.

"I think you should consider enrolling at UCLA as a psychology major."

"Really! And how am I supposed to earn a living? I have to work, you know."

"You can work here."

"Okay, now this is a joke, right?"

"Nope. I mean it. You can work here as a psychiatric aide. You'd be on the lowest rung of the ladder, but it's a great place to learn. We're looking for people to hire. You could work days and go to school at night."

"You would trust me to work here?"

"Yes, I would, with no problem."

"Have you talked to my doctor about this?"

"Yes. He thinks it's okay if you want to do it."

"Just okay?"

"He thinks it's worth a try. Psychiatrists are not the most adventuresome thinkers in the world, but he didn't say no."

"What about the medical directors, Dr. Hayman and Dr. McDowell?"

"They think it's all right. They're willing to take my word for it that you would do fine."

"I don't know about this, Don. I'm going to have to think about it."

"Right. Think about it and tomorrow we'll talk again."

I consulted Dorothy. She quickly said she thought I was a sensitive listener and I had a sharp mind. She thought I would make a good psychologist, and she had already talked to Don about it. "Do it!" she said enthusiastically. I was very flattered. The next day I talked to Dr. Feldman.

"Do you want to do this?" he asked.

"I don't know. I'm not even sure what it means."

"It means a new kind of challenge, studying hard, applying yourself, but you should only do it if it interests you."

"Yes, I think it does."

"How do you feel about working here?"

"Well, that excites me. I'd like it, I think, but it seems a little crazy, no pun intended."

"Your decision."

"I'd like to try it."

"Good. I'll sign you out so you can leave tomorrow, and I'll see you in my office at the regular time next week." He smiled as he touched my arm. "Happy New Year."

"I'm beginning to think it could be. Happy New Year to you."

I could hardly believe this was happening. I can hardly believe even now that it did happen, but it did, just this way. Christmas week, 1951, I took a giant step forward into the rest of my life.

8

Everything is changing. I am a student living in a tiny one-room studio near UCLA, a charming garden apartment building, mostly graduate students, doors ajar, an invitation to enter, talk, drink wine, share a meal, instant friends, a new life. The bookstore is gone, stock and furnishings sold. I am relieved, a burden lifted. It's good to be back in school. I feel intellectually awake and with a direction. I have my bearings again.

Don Babbidge has kept his word. Just after school starts I become a staff member at the Westerly. It seems strange at first. I still feel somewhat like a patient, but I wear a white jacket and I have in my pocket the one thing that really distinguishes me from the patients: a set of keys. It takes some getting used to.

My first few weeks I am on overload, discovering a lot about the Westerly I didn't know. Nearly all of the referring doctors and nursing staff were trained at the famous Menninger Clinic in Topeka, Kansas, where, I learn, psychoanalytic theory dictates how the hospital is run and the therapeutic approach to each patient. While not formally a teaching hospital, the Westerly is a great place to learn because everyone is enthusiastic about his or her work and equally eager to talk about it.

I attend daily shift-change and staff meetings, so I hear a lot about the rationale behind patient decisions. I love it, absorbing information like mad, my curiosity working overtime.

The job involves some duties that I can't believe I am mastering. I learn how to physically subdue an out-of-control patient, how to apply restraints, and how to roll a person in a "cold wet sheet pack," used to calm agitated patients (no pharmaceuticals for patient management yet). I am disturbed by some of the things I see and have to do, but as my identity shifts increasingly from patient to staff member, a certain distancing occurs. The madness of others is not my madness. I can approach patients with my own identity intact.

In my third month, I am sent to observe an electroshock treatment. I guess I am doing okay or they wouldn't expose me to this procedure so

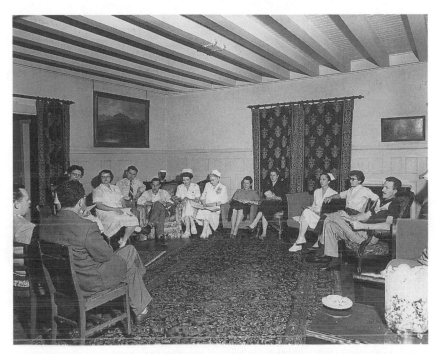

A staff meeting at the Westerly Sanitarium. I am second from the right, next to Don Babbidge, administrative director, the man who unexpectedly offered me a job in the hospital where I had been a patient.

soon. I try not to think about how narrowly I escaped this fate. I learn that electroshock is the treatment of choice for depression in most psychiatric facilities. It is not known why electroshock seems to help make a patient more available for psychotherapy. There are theories but no real understanding of the effects of running electricity through a human being's brain to artificially induce a grand mal seizure. That lack of understanding, however, does not seem to deter the use of convulsive therapy.

Inevitably, my time comes to serve on an electroshock team. Unlike Resthaven, where patients stood in line to receive their treatments, fully awake, Westerly patients are protected from even seeing the equipment. The treatments are given in the patient's private room. The cart is kept in the hall while the patient is administered a fast-acting sedative, after which the equipment is wheeled in. The electrodes are affixed to the patient's temples and held in place with a rubber headpiece. Four staff members assume their positions, one holding the shoulders from behind, two on each side, and one holding the ankles. The doctor dials up the current. The idea is to gently restrain the body as it goes through the tonic and clonic phases of the convulsion. The whole procedure is over in minutes, the equipment is wheeled out, and the patient awakens with no memory of the treatment.

The first time I was actually asked to participate, I was terrified. There is something about being in contact with those flailing arms and legs that is scary. Will I be able to function? I am determined that I will, no matter what. I am assigned to the ankles, the position that requires the least strength. I dutifully take my place. The doctor dials up the current, the patient's body goes rigid, then the jerking begins. My only thought is to apply just the right amount of pressure to the ankles to avoid broken bones. My arms move with the patient's movements. It seems to go on forever, but actually it is over quite quickly. The equipment is whisked away and the team departs. I've survived. I performed my job. I am proud of myself.

As the months go by, I am intrigued by the different states of being I observe among the Westerly patients. There are those whose lives have been disrupted by crisis and are in a process of reorganization. There are alcoholics just drying out (several movie stars among them) and some deeply into treatment and recovery from their alcoholism. Because recreational drugs are not in vogue yet, only the occasional doctor and nurse are strung out on prescription medications. There are patients severely depressed and suicidal, those who are delusional, who hallucinate, who speak in unrecognizable word salads, who walk around laughing all the time, who are mute and unmoving, who are angry and violent.

As I rotate through the wards, I come into contact with the many variations in form that mental illness can take. It is an unnerving but enlightening experience seeing how far back one can regress, how anguishing it is not to have the protection of one's defenses, how lost to the shared symbols of communication people can become. I feel the frustration of trying to connect with people who have no interest in connecting with me, or anyone.

I am occasionally asked to monitor a seclusion room, which means standing outside the heavy metal door and peering through its tiny window. When agitated patients are completely out of control and not responding to any other effort to manage them, they are isolated in this padded cell until they become more tractable. The patients are nude. They spend their time either ramming themselves against the walls, pacing in a circle, or rolled tightly into the fetal position on the floor. In the seclusion room, patients look the most like what we think of as "crazy"—all controls gone, no regard for even the appearance of rationality. It is upsetting to watch. Looking through that little window I feel as though I am party to a terrible lapse in the covenant that preserves every human being's right to dignity, no matter how far from the accepted norms of behavior he or she may have strayed. I have to remember that I am there to protect these patients from self-injury, for human beings are rarely so clever as when they are trying to destroy themselves.

There are certain places in the hospital where I am not allowed to go unless accompanied by a male aide. These are the danger zones where violent, unpredictable patients are housed. I am also warned about catatonics, cautioned never to take their immobilized state as meaning they can't spring into action at a moment's notice. I am warned, but I learn the hard way.

One day another aide, Doris, and I were feeding a catatonic woman. We were talking, being discreet, well aware that the patient probably understood everything we were saying, but I apparently had said something that didn't sit well. As we turned to leave, I heard a rustling sound behind me. I whirled around but not fast enough. The patient was out of bed, her hands around my throat, pulling me down to the floor. I felt her thumbs pressing against my windpipe as I struggled to get free.

Doris got behind the patient, grabbed her around her waist, and pulled hard. The patient lost her grip on me and was swung back onto the bed. I lay on the floor gasping for air, too frightened to speak. Doris leaned over and whispered in my ear, "Tell her you're sorry if you offended her. You've made contact with her—and that's good."

The last thing in the world I wanted to do was apologize to this person who had just nearly killed me, but I did as I was told. I stood beside the bed and said the words. The patient was silent, as immobilized as she was before. There was one difference. Her eyes locked onto mine, and the intensity of her gaze amazed me. In that moment I had a glimmer of the critical task of making contact with the severely mentally ill. It is to overcome one's own fear enough to accept any invitation such patients offer to enter their private world.

That incident was also the beginning of my understanding the therapeutic value of apologizing when you have made a mistake or when the patient thinks you have. There is a potent message in apology. It says, "I care about what happens between us and I take your feelings seriously." For many people, parental misdeeds resonate throughout their lives because no one ever said, "I'm sorry I did that to you," no one ever apologized.

In my second year at the Westerly I was allowed to participate in the staffing of patients, the discussions that shape patients' treatment plans. I had made the transition by then. I rarely ever identified with patients as I had in the beginning. I was hooked, intellectually and emotionally, on being the professional helper.

This period of learning was the most potent of my life. It gave me a sense of the mind's reach in a way that nothing else I was ever to study would. I believe that every person who practices psychotherapy should spend some time working with severely disturbed patients in order to gain a perspective on the mind's rockiest terrain and to understand how lost on that landscape one can become.

In late 1953, two years after I began work at the Westerly, the bomb fell. The hospital had to close because the low staff-to-patient ratio and the elaborate treatment plans favored by the ambitious Menninger-trained doctors were turning out to be financially too draining. I was in shock. What would the patients do? What would I do? The answer to both questions came quickly.

The medical directors had devised a plan whereby the very disturbed patients would be transferred to another hospital, but those who could be sustained at home would do so under the care of Westerly staff members, hired by the patients' families, and supervised by the attending doctor. Thus began a period of a different kind of learning—managing a patient outside the hospital environment, focusing on one person at a time, and working directly under the supervision of a psychiatrist.

I spent five days a week with a woman who was psychotic. I'll call her Ruby. When Ruby first arrived at the hospital, she was delusional and hallucinating. Because she was so unpredictable, she was placed in a glass-walled observation room next to the nurses' station so she could be watched twenty-four hours a day. Periodically Ruby would try to kill herself by climbing up on her bed, removing her nightgown, twisting it around her neck, and holding the loose end straight up over her head. She would stand this way, waiting to die, until someone went in to "cut her down."

Over the year she had been hospitalized and after many shock treatments, Ruby got better. Her behavior normalized and she graduated out of her glass-walled cage. Because of the progress she'd made, Ruby was a good candidate for the experimental release program. She had a devoted husband, no children, and an excellent psychiatrist whom she saw three times a week and with whom I consulted once a week.

Each morning, five days a week, I went to the large, luxurious apartment Ruby shared with her husband. On her good days we went out to lunch, to the movies, bowling, or shopping. On her bad days we retreated to her apartment and avoided the frightening, perilous world. Ruby particularly liked talking to people, and she took the opportunity to talk to strangers everywhere we went. They were usually drawn in because she seemed so sweet and innocent, but when Ruby moved on to asking startlingly personal questions, her victims beat a hasty retreat. At first I tried to stop these forays, but soon I decided to use them as opportunities to help Ruby distinguish what was appropriate from that which was inappropriate. I was learning to do more with bizarre behavior than just to try to stop it.

On one such occasion, I nearly lost Ruby. It was a clear, sunny Southern California day. We were out for a ride and I had the top down on my Buick convertible. I looked over at Ruby. She was smiling and seemed quite happy. Suddenly, a cat darted directly into the path of the car. There was no way to avoid hitting it, and it was immediately clear that the impact had killed it. Ruby screamed, stood up, and began climbing into the backseat, on her way out of the rear of the car. I grabbed her arm as she clambered past me, and I held on for dear life as I tried to steady my careening automobile.

"We have to get it! We have to get it," Ruby was shouting.

"Ruby, sit down! Sit down!" I shouted back.

When I was finally able to bring the car to a stop, my only concern was for my psychotic patient who was still standing up in the back seat. In as calm a voice as I could muster, I said, "Ruby, we didn't mean to do that. It was an accident. We're very sorry that it happened."

Ruby just glared at me.

"It's okay for you to feel bad about it," I said. "I feel bad too. We can talk about how we feel, but you have to stay in the car. You have to sit down in the car now."

Ruby continued to glare at me as she climbed back into the front seat and sat down.

"Why did you do that?" she asked in a hurt voice.

"It couldn't be avoided. It was an accident. It wasn't anybody's fault. It just happened. Now we have to go on and do what we were going to do, even though we feel bad. Can you do that?"

"Can *you?*" she asked.

"Yes, I can."

Ruby tossed her head back and pointed her chin straight out. "Then I can too," she said with bravado. "Let's go"

I had grown quite fond of Ruby, but after six months of the day-to-day with her, I began to feel worn out. I was invested in her recovery, but that had its downside because I was starting to feel irritated with her for not recovering more quickly. That was a sure sign that it was time for me to move on. Her psychiatrist agreed. Some years later I was delighted to hear that Ruby was in full remission and living a normal life.

My next job came through the Hacker Clinic, a Beverly Hills facility known for its celebrity clients. This time my charge was the eight-year-old daughter of a well-known movie and television star who was concerned about the effect his recent divorce from her mother was having on his daughter. The father took a house for the summer in Malibu Colony, an exclusive enclave whose residents read like a Who's Who of show business. I lived in the house with the father, the daughter, a housekeeper, and a cook. I was, ostensibly, the governess with nothing to do but spend time with my charge.

The father was a pleasant, unpretentious man, always respectful and polite to me. We had long talks and went out to dinner with his daughter and his new girlfriend, who later became his wife. It was a delicious summer, swimming, playing on the beach, more like a vacation than a job. The Colony was full of children, including the large Farrow clan two doors away. Every day I would pile Colony kids into my convertible for a ride up to the ice cream stand on the highway, where with a whoop and a holler they would all descend on the order window shouting out what they wanted.

This role was a very different one for me, relating to children. The lives of these happy, healthy Colony kids broadened my perspective on childhood. My own memories of being a child seemed far afield from who these exuberant youngsters cavorting on the beach were. By the end of the summer my charge and I had talked at length about her parents' divorce. Those bits of behavior that her father worried might be signs of disturbance had disappeared. She returned to school and her mother's home, and I returned to reality—my tiny studio apartment far from the sparkling sands of Malibu.

I liked working with children and took another assignment involving two boys, eight and twelve, whose young mother had recently died of cancer. The family lived in a Beverly Hills mansion, again complete with housekeeper and cook. I appeared five days a week, mainly to be with the eight-year-old, Michael, when he came home from school. I ate dinner with the family every night, a very formal affair, heavy oak double doors kept closed until dinner was announced, a button under the father's right foot with which to summon the staff to table. After dinner, I bathed Michael and stayed with him until he fell asleep, rubbing his forehead as his mother used to do.

Michael had a rascally sense of humor. The first night I supervised his before-bed bath, he challenged me. "I'll bet I can do something you can't do."

"I'm sure you can," I answered.

I had no warning. Michael placed his forefinger under his left eyeball and flicked. The eyeball flew across the room and landed in my lap, staring up at me. I wanted to shriek, but didn't. Michael was convulsed with laughter. "I told you I could do something you couldn't do."

"You were certainly right about that," I said, staring at his empty eye socket.

Michael's laughter subsided. "Give it back," he demanded. "C'mon, pick it up. It won't bite you."

Gingerly, I picked up the eyeball and handed it back to Michael, he deftly popped it in place, and said, "Okay, you can wash my back now."

"My, my," I thought, "wouldn't it have been nice if Michael's father had told me he had a prosthetic eye?"

Michael talked about his mother, frequently with tears. I held and comforted him. I knew he would be all right because he gave in to his grief so easily. It was Paul I was worried about because he never talked about his mother or his feelings. I wondered how much his father's stern ideas about social conduct were affecting Paul's ability to be spontaneously emotional. Even with consultation from the Hacker Clinic I was unable to break through to Paul. I had to settle for a pleasant but superficial relationship with him.

Over the year that I spent with these two boys I grew quite fond of them, so I was taken by surprise when their father announced that my job was over because they were going away for the summer. Had I thought I was going to be a permanent part of this family? Here was my first opportunity to deal with separating from individuals with whom I'd developed an emotionally intense working relationship. Nobody told me about this part. I felt bereft, like I was being left behind.

Thus began my introduction to one of the occupational hazards of working therapeutically with people. The therapist enters someone's life in a profound way for a period of time, then it's over and the client is gone. The tie is broken. The therapist has no further claim on clients, no information about them—where they are, how they are doing, what is happening to them.

I have through the years developed the appropriate clinical objectivity about all this, but I still do wonder about many of the people I have worked with. I wonder if Michael and Paul would remember me from that long-ago year of their childhood. I have them fixed in my mind as the children they were, though by now they would have their own grandchildren. Sometimes I have a whimsical fantasy about the people I have been so close to and will never see again. I see myself opening my front door, stepping out, and shouting on the wind to all of them: "Call home!"

Since leaving the Westerly as a patient, I had remained in touch with Dorothy Comingore, the actress who was largely responsible, I think, for my being talked into studying psychology. In the spring of 1952, Dorothy made good on her promise to take me to meet someone very important to her when she and I both got out of "the booby hatch," as she called it.

It was a lovely, sunny Southern California Sunday. As we drove toward Santa Monica Canyon, Dorothy explained who Salka Viertel was. She had been an actress and writer in Europe and had once been Max Reinhardt's mistress. She later married the German director Berthold Viertel and came to Hollywood with him in 1929. She met Greta Garbo then and became her great friend and confidante. Salka subsequently wrote or cowrote a number of Garbo's films, including *Anna Karenina, Queen Christina,* and *Camille.*

Salka Viertel was the grand dame of the Hollywood intelligentsia, and invitations to her Sunday-afternoon salons in Santa Monica Canyon were much sought after. The mother of three sons—Peter and Hans, both writers, and her youngest, Tom, just out of university—Salka was also the matriarch of a vital part of the Hollywood intellectual community, people young and old sought her advice and guidance.

"Having Salka's approval is very important to a lot of people in this town," Dorothy told me.

When we arrived at the big, rambling house on Maybery Road, several dozen people were already there. As we worked our way slowly through the room I could see a handsome white-haired woman at the far end surrounded by a group of people who were intently focused on what she was saying. Dorothy moved us to this circle. She greeted Salka and introduced me. Salka took my hand and seemed to study my face with great interest, but she said nothing. After a minute, she nodded as though she had completed her inspection and was delivering her verdict. It seemed to be positive. Letting go of my hand, she smiled and said, "We are always glad to meet any of Dorothy's friends. Please enjoy yourself." With that, she returned to her court.

Dorothy whispered in my ear, "She likes you." I wondered what there was to like since all I had said was "Hello."

More people arrived and the room was abuzz with conversation, a mix of languages being spoken. Dorothy gave me a running account of who was who and what they were famous for. Suddenly, startlingly, as though by a signal, all conversation came to a dead stop. Everyone's eyes turned to the stairway where a young, blonde, very svelte Shelley Winters was slowly descending, wearing a full-length mink coat on this warm day in May. Dorothy whispered in my ear that Shelley was Salka's houseguest. I remembered reading that Shelley Winters had just married the Italian actor, Vittorio Gassman, and was living in Europe.

Shelley was glamour itself as she paused dramatically on the landing, turned, and peered coquettishly over her shoulder. She then turned again and, ignoring the rest of the room, addressed Salka, speaking in a surprisingly little-girl voice, "Oh Salka, is it all right? Vittorio gave it to me."

All heads turned to Salka. "Yes, dear, it's just fine," Salka said with a smile. Shelley turned and disappeared up the stairs. The buzz of conversation resumed.

I was feeling quite comfortable at this party, accepted, attended to. I had been smiled upon by Salka Viertel, and her son, Tom Viertel, asked me out to dinner. I felt as though I had scored a home run, and I had Dorothy to thank again.

In the fall of 1952, I enrolled in a UCLA psychology course called Group Dynamics, taught by Dr. Evelyn Hooker, a tall, imposing woman with a deeply resonant voice and a commanding presence. I was fascinated by her lectures on why people behaved as they did in small groups. The second hour of the class was a laboratory session in which we were to experience in small groups the processes Dr. Hooker had talked about in her lectures.

Unexpectedly, I immediately became the leader of my group, surprising because I had gone all through college without ever once raising my hand or speaking in class because I was shy. But something happened in that group that tapped into a strength I didn't know I had. I continued to lead the group throughout the semester. A spark was ignited. I knew somehow that studying and leading groups was going to become a major focus of my professional life. It is ironic that this important learning experience happened with Evelyn Hooker, who would come into my life often in later years in ways wholly unrelated to group dynamics.

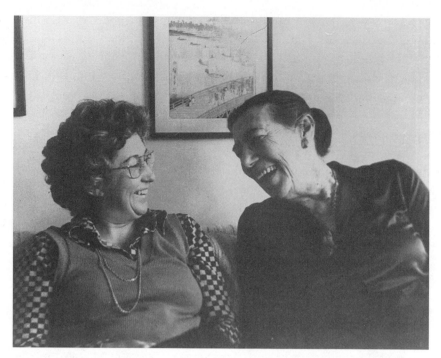

Dr. Evelyn Hooker at her Santa Monica apartment in the 1970s. She had been my teacher at UCLA in the 1950s and she continued to be in my life as a friend. I presented her at the first symposium UCLA ever did on homosexuality.

Dr. Evelyn Hooker was a social psychologist who would later become famous in her field for ground-breaking research on the mental health of homosexual men. First presented at a meeting of the American Psychological Association in the summer of 1956, her finding that homosexuality is a "sexual pattern which is within the normal range, psychologically," marked a turning point in the way homosexuality would be viewed and studied forever after.

In 1952 Dr. Hooker was already informally collecting data from gay men, but very few people knew about it. She would not begin systematic gathering of data until two years later, and it would not be until the 1960s that her landmark work would attract widespread attention. Our paths would cross again in the early 1970s when I coordinated the first day-long seminar on homosexuality at UCLA; Evelyn Hooker was one of my panel members. In 1979, she wrote the introduction to the first edition of my book *Positively Gay*, having become by then the internationally renowned expert in the field. In the early 1950s, ironically though, it was not her studies on sexuality that drew us together but her teaching on the process by which small groups function.

During these years in the 1950s I essentially purged homosexuality from my life. Lila had returned to New York, so I no longer had contact with the lesbians who were her friends. I knew a few gay men, but I believed their sexuality had nothing to do with me. I dated men, although I was wary about becoming emotionally entangled with anybody. Dr. Feldman was pleased that I was dating men. He periodically reassured me that I was not homosexual, and I felt bolstered by his confidence.

Did Fred Feldman do me a disservice by reinforcing my own homophobia? Given the zeitgeist of the 1950s, I don't see how he could have done anything different. If he had supported my homosexuality, he would have been encouraging what he believed to be pathological. I have never wavered in my certainty that his only motive was to help me. I'm just sorry that he didn't stick around to see the world change. I truly believe he would have changed with it. In later years, I wanted to go back to Dr. Feldman for two reasons: to fix his thinking about homosexuality and gay people and to pay him something for the years he saw me without charge. I was distressed to learn he had died before I could reconnect with him. I still believe I owe him my life.

Having finished my undergraduate studies in 1955, I decided to take a break from being a full-time student. I'd heard that the Military Hospital Service of the American Red Cross offered possibilities for travel abroad. I had no idea what military life was about, it just seemed like an adventure, something different to do, and I was ready for something different. I signed up and was sent to Oak Knoll Naval Hospital in Oakland for six weeks of training on military etiquette, hospital routines, and what the American Red Cross is *not* about, for instance, selling coffee on the battlefield, a ridiculous old rumor that the ARC had to continually refute.

Uniformed down to the regulation hat and shoes, I was posted to the 3275th U.S. Air Force Hospital at Parks Air Force Base in Pleasanton, California, where oddly enough there was no airstrip and there were no airplanes. Parks was a training base and home to a thousand-bed hospital where I was assigned as a recreation worker.

I quickly learned some things about the military scene that had not been taught at Oak Knoll. For instance, sex was an integral part of military life. I was assigned to a mixed bachelor officer quarters (BOQ). The men lived downstairs and the women—nurses, officers, and Red Cross workers—lived upstairs. The twain often met in the common room downstairs where the nightly parties occurred. The flirting usually started during the cocktail hour and inevitably turned into musical beds later in the evening.

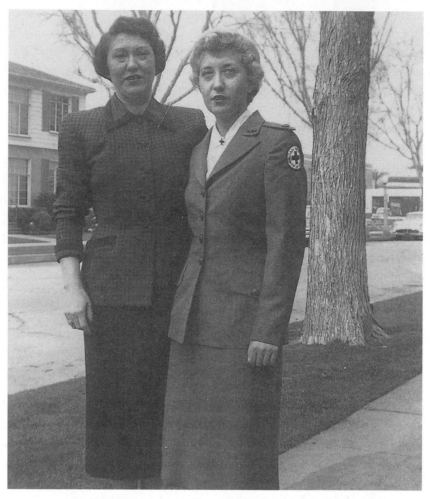

Visiting my mother in 1956. I am in uniform, a case worker in the
Military Hospital Service of the American Red Cross.

The only people who did not join the party were certain inhabitants of
the second floor who, I was quite sure, were lesbians. They were female
Red Cross workers older than the twenty- and thirty-something nurses and
officers, and they tended to keep very much to themselves. Needless to say,
I gave them a wide berth, having carefully established my heterosexual cre-
dentials by nonstop involvement in the parties downstairs.

My initial assignment as a recreation worker was to run the hospital servicemen's club, where ambulatory patients gathered to play pool or watch
television. I quickly learned that the troublemakers in a peacetime military

hospital were the young orthopedic patients injured in car crashes, usually because they were driving drunk. They were the juvenile delinquents of the hospital culture.

My introduction to the troublemakers, and to a very crucial aspect of military discipline, came on the first Sunday night I was on duty alone in the service club. Around 7 P.M., a sudden influx of orthopedic patients returned from their weekend passes. It took me a few minutes to realize that most of them were drunk. I didn't see what started it, but within a very short time a fight began and the entire room erupted in violence. Crutches were flying, fists smashing into bodies, leg casts used to kick, blood on the walls. I watched in horror, stunned and immobilized. Then I woke up—I was in charge, I had to do something. Pulling myself up to my full five feet, I shouted, "Stop this! Stop this minute!" No one even looked in my direction.

I retreated to my office and quickly dialed the Officer of the Day. Minutes later the O.D. arrived. He stopped cold in the doorway and surveyed the wild scene—patients slamming against one another, being shoved into walls, obscenities filling the air. The O.D. moved forward a few steps, took a deep breath, and roared, "'TENSHUN!"

To my utter amazement, everything stopped, everyone in the room froze and snapped to attention. I couldn't believe it. The O.D. began barking orders. He lined up the injured against one wall and everybody else against another. He had each patient shout out his name and ward number, which he duly recorded. Then he ordered certain of the uninjured to escort the wounded to the emergency room and everyone else to return to their ward. The patients moved with dispatch.

Only minutes before, this room had been in chaos. I understood immediately the meaning of military discipline—unquestioning obedience to unchallenged authority. It is the hedge against disaster, the ability to redirect behavior in an instant, perhaps making the difference between life and death. Days, weeks, months of training and in a split second it is all brought to bear. I understood even more the next day when I came upon a dozen of the previous night's rioters on their hands and knees meticulously scrubbing the front steps of the hospital with toothbrushes, inch by inch, discipline reinforced by humility. How dehumanizing military life could be, how efficiently it all worked.

A few months later I had a new assignment that was less turbulent but much more challenging. Parks Air Force Hospital had five full wards of tuberculosis patients, young men who had been diagnosed early through routine x-rays. They felt healthy but were considered highly contagious. The treatment of choice in 1955 was bed rest, twelve to eighteen months confined to a ward. These young men were robust, restless, bored, and resentful, living in one long room, bed after bed, with no way to escape one another. When I arrived, the main focus of activity was on the huge brightly lit tanks of fighting fish on each ward. The patients would gather round the tanks cheering on their favorite combatants as each ferocious battle was played out.

It was almost by accident that I came upon the activity that was to be my success story on the tuberculosis service. One night I brought a phonograph and a stack of records to the wards. I had just taken a course on the history of jazz at UCLA, and I used my notes to talk about the background of each piece we heard and how it fit into the story of the development of jazz in this country. The patients loved it. I brought them books to read on the subject, and soon there were discussion groups.

I wrote to Nesuhi Ertegan of Atlantic Records, Ahmet's brother and my jazz teacher at UCLA, asking for records, and he sent cartonfuls. He also sent my letter on to the editors of *Downbeat* and *Metronome,* and they printed my appeal, which brought more records. A Bay Area disc jockey, Pat Henry, invited me to his studio to borrow records every week. Ralph Gleason, the San Francisco music critic, publicized our program, and it was written up in the *Army Times* and the *Oakland Tribune.*

The patients put together a jazz hour that was broadcast daily over the hospital radio station, and they started the Parks Air Force Base Jazz Club. They designed stationery and began to correspond with jazz clubs all over the world. Hospital staff said they had never seen TB patients so involved in anything. I wrote a report of what I had done so that other Red Cross recreation workers could start jazz clubs in their military hospitals.

I felt very fulfilled by this work and was confident that the jazz program would continue without me when I was reassigned to the Army Hospital at Fort Ord in Monterey. I had completed the educational requirements and was being promoted to caseworker, a much more sedate job, though it too had its perils.

During my first week at Fort Ord I had to inform a young serviceman and his wife that their three-year-old daughter had died. As gently as I could, I told them what had happened. Feeling near tears myself, I handed them the brown paper bag that contained their child's tiny clothes and shoes. The mother took the shoes out of the bag and turned them over and over in her hands, silently, as if in a trance. Her husband led her out of the room. I heard her scream in the hallway. I didn't sleep that night.

In the middle of dinner one evening that same week, I was called to the operating room to interview a woman in the throes of a bloody miscarriage. My job was to get information and do something about the five small children she had left unattended at home. I never got back to the dining room.

To offset the more unsettling aspects of being a hospital caseworker, I bought a little English sports car and joined the Pebble Beach Sports Car Club. I loved the rallies and racing along the beach roads with the top down. One day at a rally I met a tall, handsome soldier named Bill. Soon Bill was driving my sports car in the rallies. He ran the hospital radio station and, like me, he lived in the hospital compound. We dated and had a lot of fun together with "our" sports car. I was never quite sure if it was me or my car that Bill was attracted to until he, about to be discharged from the Army, surprised me by asking me to marry him.

Bill had a wonderful life programmed for us. His parents would spring for a house in the suburbs as a wedding present, he was already accepted in a corporate executive training program, we would raise kids and live the American dream. I was flattered. After all, this was what I wanted, to be married, have a family, but as I listened to Bill describe our future, it had a stifling, airless feel about it. Maybe I just wasn't that attracted to him, maybe I wasn't ready for so planned out a life, so constricting a scenario, one that was more about him than me. I politely declined his proposal. Sometimes the dream turns on itself when it collides with reality. I wanted so much to marry, but when presented with the possibility, I backed off— not yet, not right, not ready.

The Army hospital at Fort Ord was a community unto itself. The huge complex had it all—movie theaters, all kinds of shops, cafes, bars, a ready-made social life. One never had to leave the base. Toward the end of 1957 I began to realize that I was basically losing touch with the outside world. I had become institutionalized, totally immersed in military life. It was time to get off the reservation and back into civilian life.

I took a job as a probation officer with the San Diego County Probation Department. My work was with delinquent girls and dependent children who had been abused or neglected. Working with delinquent teenagers in the 1950s was a walk in the park compared to what it later became. We dealt with rebellious antics and minor infractions of the law, nothing very serious. The decade was a time of innocence absent the anger that later came to permeate the minds and hearts of disadvantaged youth in a society that didn't seem to give a damn about them. Drugs were not yet at the center of kids' lives. Guns had not yet turned the streets into killing fields.

My supervisor in the probation department was a lovely woman named Mrs. Creel. She was a model of refinement, a dainty, delicate, elegant little person who seemed totally out of place in the down-and-dirty world of teenage delinquency, abusive parents, and neglected children. She had been at it for many years, however, and knew it all. One day I went to Mrs. Creel with a problem that I was certain I had acquired in the line of duty.

"I think I have crabs."

Mrs. Creel fixed me with a vaguely pained look.

"I'm sure I got them when I packed Jackie's underwear to take her to Juvenile Hall. The staff there told me she came in with crabs."

Mrs. Creel said in a quiet voice, "*Pediculosis pubis.*"

"What?"

"*Pediculosis pubis.* That's the proper name for what you have."

"What do I do about it?"

"A-200," she said without expression.

"What's that?"

"That's what you apply to the affected area after you've shaved it."

"I have to *shave* it?"

"Daily."

"My god! Daily?"

Mrs. Creel nodded, her eyes intent now on the papers she was shuffling.

"How long will it take to get rid of my . . . *pediculosis?*"

Mrs. Creel looked up at me, peering over the little gold half-glasses that sat on her nose. Words were not needed. This discussion was clearly at an end.

During the two years I worked as a probation officer, my personal life was more peaceful and uncomplicated than it had ever been. I lived at the beach, partied, learned to sail, dated men, and took university extension classes at night. It was in one of those classes that my life would be transformed for the next decade.

9

Dick Farson was a tall, extraordinarily handsome man. He had a rugged face and a great jutting jaw with a Cary Grant cleft in the middle of his chin. He looked like a movie star, and it was difficult not to keep looking at him.

"Are you bored?" he asked.

It took a few seconds for me to realize that Farson was talking to me. Flustered, I stammered, "Uh, no. What do you mean?"

"When someone in my class opens a book and starts reading while I'm lecturing, I assume they are bored."

I had no answer.

"What do you think of what I've been talking about?"

"It's . . . uh . . . interesting."

I'd registered for Client-Centered Therapy, a class about an alternative approach to psychotherapy that put emphasis on the relationship between therapist and client rather than theories about the client's pathology. I'd chosen this class particularly because it was taught by this instructor, a protégé of Carl Rogers. Rogers was a giant figure in the field of psychology and the inventor of the client-centered approach to psychotherapy. Although I was genuinely interested in the subject matter, this instructor seemed terribly full of himself, arrogant, and glib, so I decided I didn't like him and I would drop the course. That's when I opened the book. Farson was still looking at me. I had to say something. "Well, I don't think I'll take this course after all. I was just waiting for the break to leave."

"Thank you," he said, "at least that's honest." Then his voice took on the seductive tone that I was to hear many times in the years ahead. "I hope you don't leave." His face softened and he flashed his Cary Grant smile. Why was he was going to so much trouble to hold onto one student—and why me? I closed my book. He continued lecturing. I tried to look interested. I was relieved when he announced the break. Getting up to leave, I saw that he was watching me. I felt less sure now about what to do, curious about his interest in me. Breaking away from the group of students around him, he approached me.

"Decided?"

"Not yet."

"Good. Then why don't you stay?"

He stood very close and peered intently at me. I looked away from him, but I couldn't shake the awareness of his eyes on me. In that moment I sensed that something unusual was happening, and I knew I was going to do what he wanted me to do.

"Okay, I'll stay."

"Good," he said, and leaning toward me he touched me lightly on the shoulder. For the rest of the session, and the semester, I listened carefully to Dick Farson. He frequently smiled and nodded in my direction, as though to reward me for staying with him. I would later come to understand how acutely important every personal conquest was for Dick, but at the time I was simply hooked.

When the course was over, a few of us formed a study group that met weekly in Dick's office. I continued to feel that he found something special in me, but now that he really knew me I trusted the feeling more. I was reminded of the way Don Babbidge had beamed in on something in me when I was a patient at the Westerly (which seemed like a thousand years ago).

Toward the end of the summer Dick began talking enthusiastically about a research institute that he and another psychologist were starting with the backing of a wealthy benefactor. To my great surprise and delight, he offered me a job as a research assistant, also suggesting that I enroll at San Diego State University in the graduate psychology program. Of course I agreed. It was thrilling to have someone care enough about me to want to design my future.

I became the first employee of the Western Behavioral Sciences Institute, which would grow to be the one of the most important centers of behavioral science research in the world. WBSI was started in a one-bedroom suite at a La Jolla motel by the two founders, Dick Farson and Bud Crow; the benefactor, Paul Lloyd; a secretary; and me. WBSI soon moved to its own building as the staff grew, projects were funded, and visiting fellows began to arrive.

From the beginning, WBSI was on the cutting edge, supporting research that explored the potential of human beings rather than the ways we are disordered. This research was the sort that the conservative universities would never support because it was considered too "soft-minded." Though I was nominally a research assistant, Dick encouraged me to design a study of my own. His confidence in me made me feel as though I could do anything.

I had never forgotten my fascination with what I had learned about small-group process in Evelyn Hooker's UCLA class, so I designed a study that would also become my master's thesis at San Diego State, *The Influence of Residual Parental Threat on the Determination of Initiated Interaction Patterns in Group Psychotherapy;* in other words, who talked to whom in group sessions and could one predict those patterns on the basis of how similar each group member was to a parent with whom one had unfinished business? The study took two years to complete and in July 1962 was published in the *International Journal of Group Psychotherapy,* my first recognition in print. It also marked the beginning of my immersion in the research and development work that would be at the center of my work life for the next sixteen years.

While my learning experiences at WBSI were truly mind expanding, my formal graduate education at San Diego State was truly mind boggling. Getting my thesis approved became a nightmare of dealing with pompous, punitive faculty members who seemed to take delight in torturing graduate students. My committee was still diddling themselves over whether to approve my thesis months after it had been published in a prestigious international psychology journal.

Those nine years at WBSI were golden, and it was there I got my real education in psychology. Eventually I co-led groups with Dick Farson and spent many hours with him discussing the dynamics of what had occurred in the sessions. I learned research methodology from a smart, young psychologist on staff named Larry Solomon. Larry was a born teacher, and I benefited from his vast knowledge of social and clinical psychology. We later codirected several studies and edited a book together, *New Perspectives on Encounter Groups.*

Dick Farson assembled a superb board of trustees for WBSI, including his own mentor, Carl Rogers, and semanticist S. I. Hayakawa. I was allowed to sit in on the quarterly board meetings. Carl was always the voice of reason, and "Don" Hayakawa (a nickname he acquired as a "don" teaching in Canadian universities) was the conservative voice, when he was awake. His tendency to snooze during meetings earned him public ridicule many years later when he became a U.S. senator from California.

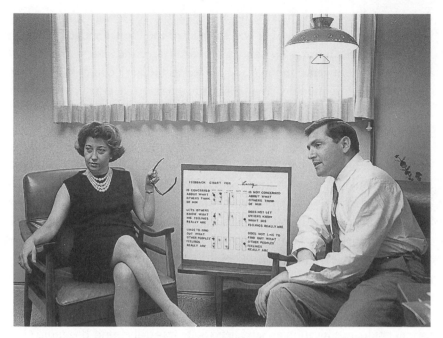

Dr. Lawrence Solomon, my colleague throughout the 1960s at the Western Behavioral Sciences Institute in La Jolla, California, where we conducted research on small group process and edited a book together, *New Perspectives on Encounter Groups,* for which Carl Rogers wrote the foreword.

WBSI grew rapidly. In 1963, Carl Rogers became a permanent resident fellow. Soon after, Abraham Maslow, the founder of humanistic psychology, became a visiting fellow, followed by Alex Bavelas, who did brilliant early work on group dynamics, Jack Gibb, a pioneer in organizational theory, the philosopher Abe Kaplan, and Ted Newcombe, known as the "father of social psychology." The fellows had only one obligation to WBSI: to discuss their work with the staff in weekly informal seminars. These sessions were unparalleled opportunities for learning. It was like having the university come to us.

Without the hoops to jump through—grades, exams, faculty approval— we were free to deal with ideas, to think creatively, to learn without having to prove ourselves. The two people who had the greatest influence on me in this period were Rogers and Maslow, both monolithic figures in modern psychology.

When Abe Maslow came to WBSI with his wife Bertha, it had been five years since he first began talking about the controversial ideas that were to become the basis for the "third force" in psychology—a reaction to the traditional approaches of Freudian psychoanalysis and classical behaviorism. Maslow's notion was that there was more to be learned about human nature from fully functioning, self-actualized people than from the psychopathology of Freud's subjects. He studied the lives of many of the great achievers of history—Einstein, Goethe, Spinoza, Lincoln, Franklin—to understand what enabled them to accomplish all they did.

While he was at WBSI, Abe Maslow was exploring "peak experiences," those times when one is able to leave all fears, doubts, and inhibitions behind to know moments of pure joy. I helped him collect data and spent many hours discussing how and why such peak experiences occurred. I felt privileged to be his sounding board, to have the gift of his time, to experience the workings of his imaginative mind one-on-one.

Abe Maslow was a tall man with a quintessentially Jewish face, a bristly mustache, and a quick smile. His voice purred when he spoke, and he loved to talk, his conversation richly textured with quotations from literature and philosophy. I became friends with Abe and Bertha, a beautiful woman, white-haired, soft, loving, who made me feel like family. I hadn't realized how WASPish WBSI was until the Maslows arrived. Before that Larry Solomon and I were the only Jewish presence.

By 1963, when Carl Rogers became a permanent fellow, he had achieved such eminence that his affiliation as a staff member catapulted WBSI into world prominence. His ideas about psychotherapy redefined for many the role of the psychotherapist, the task of the client, and the purpose of the therapeutic process. Carl was a rather ordinary-looking midwesterner with a compact muscular body, in extraordinary shape for a man in his sixties. Because he loved the outdoors, his nearly bald head was always handsomely suntanned. He had a pleasant face, but his eyes had a sad look as though he'd witnessed something that had made him forever melancholy. Carl was an inveterate memo writer. He wrote memos in which he shared his dreams for the future, his works-in-progress, and wonderful, long, colorful travelogues of his trips. Helen Rogers seemed an enigma to me; tall, large-framed, white-haired, and bespectacled, she looked stern even when she smiled. I never really got to know her, not sure where to begin with this American Gothic who, when she looked at me at all, didn't seem to actually see me.

A few years after he joined the WBSI staff, Carl Rogers established a postdoctoral fellowship program in psychotherapy to which postdocs came from all over the world. I had no strong interest at the time in becoming a therapist—I was very happily involved in research—but studying with Carl Rogers was too tempting an opportunity to pass up. Carl allowed me to sit in on the seminars and to do counseling under his supervision. In years to come I would be grateful for this extraordinary experience.

Carl was for the most part a patient and supportive teacher, but when he heard something on the tape of a therapy session that seemed to him a betrayal of a client's trust, he would hit the stop button and confront. One day my turn came:

"Why the hell are you arguing with this woman?" Carl exploded.

I hadn't realized I was.

"She is trying to tell you what she feels, and you are telling her that she's really feeling something else. *She* is the authority on how she feels, not *you*. Listen to her. Listen!" And, with that, Carl flipped the recorder back on.

My mind raced back to Dr. Feldman, who had helped me so much. Of course it wasn't his intellectual interpretations of my feelings that made the difference; it was my perception that he really heard me and cared about me. I could open up to him because I trusted his concern. Wasn't this a lesson not only about psychotherapy but about all relationships? "Don't help me," I've often wanted to say to people in my life. "Just listen and let me know you care."

Carl Rogers's work gave rise to the Human Potential Movement. Happily for me, he was very interested in the intensive group experience as a way of enabling change in people, and he acted as a consultant on all my research projects. It was Carl who gave a name to the kinds of personal growth groups that came to be at the heart of the Human Potential Movement. He called them "basic encounter groups." Encounter stuck, basic didn't.

Encounter groups are weekend or sometimes weeks-long group experiences in which eight to ten people, meeting with a facilitator, explore themselves and their interactions in an effort to improve how they function interpersonally. In the 1960s, encounter groups swept the country. They were widely reported on in the media and were sought out by hundreds of thousands of people. Carl Rogers's name was synonymous with the encounter group movement.

My own work at WBSI evolved into identifying what important conditions were absent in a personal growth group when a therapist was not present to create them. From what we learned, we developed audiotape programs to enable self-directed groups to create their own "therapeutic conditions." Our objective was to provide personal growth opportunities to large numbers of people who would not otherwise have access to such experiences. We planned to do that through the use of technology—audiotape recorders. It seems ludicrous now that tape recorders were our "high-tech" instruments, but that's what we had. The recorded tapes were the equivalent of today's software.

In the mid-1960s, my self-directed group project began to attract the attention of the national media. Featuring the unique aspect of "leaderless" personal growth groups run by tape recorders, articles appeared in the *New York Times* and other newspapers. In 1967, Walter Cronkite devoted an entire episode of his television program, *21st Century,* to my futuristic tape-led groups. Titled "Circle of Love," the CBS program followed a group of young people meeting for three days in sessions conducted by my audiotape program.

Playboy, in an article titled "Alternatives to Analysis," portrayed the possibility of millions of people going through my tape-led groups: "These millions will then reshape society into a sort of single big happy uninhibited affectionate turned-on encounter group." The author of the *Playboy* article told the story of my being stranded for three full days in the TWA terminal at JFK Airport during a fierce blizzard in the 1960s:

> Listening to the incessant bulletins over the airport loudspeakers and watching her frustrated fellow travelers grow increasingly bored and glassy-eyed, she kept grieving at the lost opportunity for playing her *Encountertapes* [as they were called by then] over the speakers and turning an ordeal into a delightful mass initiation into the marvels of the encounter group.

The truth is that I did have that fantasy, thinking about what it would be like to have ENCOUNTERTAPES broadcast over the public address system to the six thousand marooned and miserable souls wandering around that TWA terminal for three days. Organized into encounter groups, maybe they would not have been so desperate to make contact with the outside world that they worked the phones to their breaking point until the receivers of every telephone in the terminal hung limp and useless against the walls. Maybe the hungry hordes would not have assaulted and knocked unconscious the man wheeling the first cart of helicoptered-in food at the beginning of the third day, every peanut and candy bar in the place already eaten. And maybe they wouldn't have had to lock up the liquor after too many drinkers became combative and obnoxious on the second day.

Ensconced in the Ambassador's Club on the mezzanine along with the other "privileged" travelers, I looked down at the main floor where circles of students sat on blankets on the floor, talking, laughing, playing guitars, and singing. They knew how to stay in the here and now rather than obsessing about what was going on out there without them. My tape-led group sessions could have helped everyone do that, at least that was my thought as I whiled away the hours of boredom.

Actually, my fantasy about guiding thousands through a personal growth experience with my ENCOUNTERTAPE program was not so far fetched. I had already done it experimentally in a large school building with one tape recorder and one set of tapes, broadcast over the public address system. Several hundred people in small groups met in different rooms listening to the tapes that structured each of their sessions. After the heady experience of watching a mass demonstration of my work, I began to think about variations on the theme, environments in which I could promote personal growth interaction in a variety of life situations, wherever people gathered or were stuck, spending unstructured time: in emergency shelters, hospital waiting rooms, jails, airports, or train stations. I was excited by these possibilities for change. At WBSI, such thoughts were called "blue-skying," a practice that was encouraged as a way to broaden our thinking and create new challenges. It didn't take much for me to fly into the wild blue yonder. I loved playing with the future. Still do.

In 1964 I received my first research grant from the federal government to evaluate the effectiveness of tape-led therapeutic groups with vocational rehabilitation clients. I was also receiving validation within my profession by publishing papers in psychological journals and frequently presenting my work at professional meetings. But my good feelings about myself were occasionally marred by experiences that stirred the conflict inside me that I'd thought I had under control. One of Carl's postdoctoral fellows was a woman I'll call Jan. She tried very hard to get to know me even though I constantly rebuffed her. She was clearly a homosexual who didn't seem to care who knew it.

One day she came into my office and stood stiffly before my desk.

"I need to say this to you. I know you have been avoiding me and I know why. I just wonder if you know why. I think it's sad that you have to protect yourself like this. I'm not offended, because I understand. I hope that someday you will come to understand too. For now, I just feel sorry for you."

She hastily left the room. I was furious. Who did she think she was confronting me like that? How dare she presume to know more about me than I knew about myself? Damn her!

In the sleepy little town of La Jolla where I spent the 1960s, you would never know that a cultural revolution was shaking the foundations of American society. There were no hippies, love-ins, psychedelic celebrations, or demonstrations protesting the Vietnam War. La Jolla was removed from all that, a haven for affluent retirees and a beach resort where the young people were blond, tanned, and gorgeous.

Relief from the vacuousness of all this "white-bread" was the sprinkling of intellectuals attached to the Scripps Institution of Oceanography (eleven Nobel Prize winners), the Scripps Clinic, and the Salk Insititute. I gained entrance to this crowd through the volunteers at WBSI. Toni Volcani was one. Her husband, Ben, was a physicist at the Scripps Institution, and evenings at the Volcanis were always intriguing because there were sure to be at least two or three Nobel laureates present.

One night at a party at Toni's I was asked to dance by a tall, rugged Englishman with a most cheerful personality. As we were dancing I told him my name and asked his. "Frank," he said, smiling in such a way as to make me suspect this must not be his real name. After several dances, "Frank" escorted me back to my seat, where he was immediately approached by another guest, who gushed, "Sir Francis, how nice to see you!"

It took only one second for me to realize that I had been dancing with Sir Francis Crick, who had just been awarded the Nobel Prize for his part in discovering the structure of DNA, the basic building block of human life. A definite perk of the La Jolla scene was rubbing shoulders (and sometimes anything else) with such extraordinary people.

My social life was relentlessly heterosexual and altogether integrated with the activities of WBSI. As I look back on it, I see myself making an enormous effort to blend in, to be like everyone around me. All of my friends were married couples, and I essentially lived their life. I hosted and attended dinner parties, played tennis, went to the beach and the horse races, and gossiped. Even though wives tended to get a little nervous around single women who had a companionable working relationship with their husbands, I was accepted as one of the crowd. I learned the secret early, to always talk first to the wives on social occasions, seeming to be more interested in them than in their husbands.

I had a parade of male suitors with whom I diligently pursued relationships, none of which ripened into anything serious, but as long as I was involved with men I felt that I was okay. Whenever I got too close to my women friends in La Jolla, too involved or attached, I backed off, allowing myself no feelings of attraction toward women. The antidote to even hints of such feelings was always a roll in the hay with a man to demonstrate to myself that I was still normal.

I convinced myself that I really preferred sex with men, a notion that was reinforced by my therapist-of-the-moment, who encouraged accounts of satisfying heterosexual experiences for which I was usually rewarded by a nod and an approving smile. Actually, I did enjoy intimacy with many of the men I had sex with because they were attractive, decent, interesting human beings, but I also had a growing awareness that something was essentially missing.

One of the ways people deal with unacceptable aspects of their lives is to compartmentalize experiences that can then be denied as not having really happened. I did that with the periodic forays into homosexuality that I made during the 1960s, always far from home, usually in New York, never with anyone connected to my "real" life in La Jolla. In New York I had gay male friends who were forever pushing me into sexual escapades with women. *They* made me do it, I simply *cooperated.*

One weekend at a friend's country house in Connecticut, I was assigned to a bedroom with an attractive blonde Viennese woman named Schatzi. She claimed she was a countess, oft married and pursued by hordes of men. The second night of our stay in the country, she crawled into my bed. That's when I realized my gay male buddies had set us up, knowing that each of us "swung both ways," as they put it in those days. For a time, there were repeat performances with Schatzi when our travels brought us both to New York, but eventually she married again and was no longer available for our we're-not-really-lesbians lovemaking.

On other trips away from La Jolla, there was Norma, a captain in the U.S. Army. We met through a mutual gay male friend. Her masculine appearance put me off at first because there was no denying it—she was a dyke. But she was an experienced dyke, a sweet, gentle lover who knew her way around the erotic landscape and taught me ways of pleasuring I hadn't dreamed existed. When she retired from the army, she decamped to live in Europe.

On another New York trip, there was Samantha (Sammy for short), a

Broadway actress who, like the countess, had been with many men. She was quite beautiful, and I was bewitched. We spent long New York afternoons talking, in a holding pattern for sex that I didn't understand required me to be the initiator. Because I didn't understand that, we never got beyond cuddling and kissing, but I was so enamored and so flattered by her interest in me that I went back again and again just to look at her, to be touched by her. After a while she tired of my "inability to get it up," as she so delicately put it.

There were others, often found and presented to me by gay male friends at parties, alcohol easing the contact, shadowy figures with names long forgotten, my only souvenir of these encounters a feeling of disappointment in myself afterwards. I saw all this as having nothing to do with my real life. New York was a playground where my playmates were characters in a surreal drama that could be forgotten as soon as the curtain fell. I never told my therapist in La Jolla about these adventures, but I did tell him about the heterosexual flings I quickly returned to in order to demonstrate to myself, and to him, that I wasn't really gay.

As for involvements with a little more depth than the shallow reassurance I got from one-night stands, I found myself having affairs with married men. To say "I found myself" is indicative of the lack of responsibility I took for making these affairs happen. What I didn't understand at the time was how consistently safe these entanglements were. The seeds of destruction were built into every liaison I had with a man married to someone else, little chance that a satisfying relationship of my own would ever ensue.

As I think back on this period of my life I am appalled at the lack of respect I had for other people's partnerships. Such relationships had no sanctity in my mind, they were abstractions that I didn't really understand. My relationship with Luce had little grounding in reality for me, because homosexuality seemed such a shaky foundation on which to build commitment. Incredibly, it didn't enter my mind that my actions might be hurting someone else. I thought of what I was doing with married men only in terms of what I was after. What I also didn't understand was the shell game I was playing with myself, constantly switching the issues so I would never have to confront the one that scared me the most.

I met Roberto Zelaya at a party in New York in the late sixties. I don't know just what caused the spark between us, but we bonded right from the

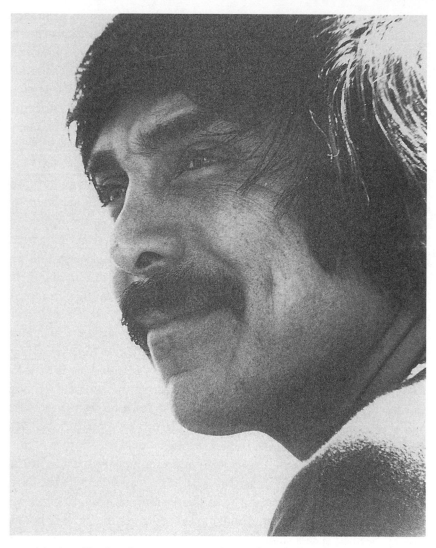

My dear friend and constant companion, Roberto Zelaya, a gay man who accompanied me to lesbian bars and tried to push me toward women, unsuccessfully.

beginning. Gay and extraordinarily handsome, he was an out-of-work actor. Unfortunately for him, Roberto was never able to overcome his heavy Honduran accent sufficiently to find success as an actor in New York. Ignoring this salient fact, in 1968 I began a campaign for him to come to Los Angeles, where I had just moved, to pursue a career in films. That of course was the surface reason. I really wanted him around me because I liked the person

I was when I was with him. He took me up on my idea, made the move, and became an indispensable part of my life.

Being with Roberto got me totally out of my serious professional self and into the part of me that I had kept a lid on for a long time, too afraid to act crazy for fear I might once again go crazy. Roberto and I were silly together. We made up outrageous scenarios and pretended we were the characters we had invented, sometimes to the embarrassment of our friends who thought we were too squirrelly.

I loved Roberto's various "looks." He could be Rudolph Valentino sloe-eyed seductive or a little boy prankster, merry eyes sparkling with mischief. Although he was gay (I wasn't, of course) and more than ten years my junior, we had a wonderfully romantic relationship. We held hands and held each other, intimate, loving, sensual, and sometimes even sexual. We were an odd couple whose lives had intersected and become hooked into one another.

The 1960s shattered the status quo. From the death of John F. Kennedy, the first walk on the moon, and the Vietnam War to the black and women's movements, and the sexual revolution, it was a decade of enormous upheaval and change. African Americans were finding their collective voice to say to white America, "We've had enough of being defined by you, of being told where we can and can't go. We know what's possible, and we see the power in ourselves to achieve it. The time for change is now."

The success of the Civil Rights Movement in gaining the attention of the country inspired other groups historically discriminated against to begin to think and act in more self-determining ways. Stirred by the challenges to tradition that were going on all around them, young people were becoming increasingly disaffected by middle-class values. The country was practically under siege from the various liberation movements that were dismantling convention and exploring new ways of being in the world.

Bob Dylan sounded the call to arms: "Everybody must get stoned!" The alteration in consciousness that has had the most profound effect on American life came with the introduction of mind-altering drugs to the youth of the country in the 1960s. Marijuana, long a staple of the jazz world, was just beginning to find its way onto college campuses and into the streets of large cities where young people were gathering to play out a crisis of identity that was to last for an entire decade and more.

Experimentation didn't stop with marijuana. LSD was extolled as the miracle fix for the New Age. Hope is just another hit away! The quest for magic potions that has followed on these early, innocent forays into drug use has become awesomely destructive. The new business of illicit drugs took shape and an international killer industry was born. America has never been the same since.

While La Jolla was not exactly psychedelically inclined, it would have been difficult for anyone under forty to get through the sixties without some involvement with drugs. I learned early on that I was extremely sensitive to most mind-altering substances. I hallucinated on marijuana, sufficiently to scare me off it. I never graduated to anything more psychoactive than pot until twenty years later when I attended board meetings of a prestigious gay organization where after-meeting socializing routinely featured the 1980s drug of choice, cocaine.

"Try it. Try it. C'mon. You'll love it!" The dollar bills were rolled, the lines laid out, and I was implored to join the party. Okay. I'll try it. I snorted a line, I felt the rush, and I loved it. I did another line, then stopped, but everyone else kept going. Months later, at the next meeting, I snorted again and loved it even more. I decided to buy some to take back to Los Angeles with me. I was nervous about carrying it on the airplane, so a fellow board member offered to carry it if I would give her some of it.

At home I anticipated with delight the feeling I knew I would get from the cocaine hit. I got out the little container of white powder and rolled it around in my hand, previewing the pleasurable sensations to come. Then, suddenly, my thoughts shifted to a disturbing idea—I could get into this habit very easily. I thought about clients whose lives had been blighted by the escalating use of cocaine. I thought about the brilliant friend I recently visited on the psychiatric ward at Cedars-Sinai recovering from his cocaine addiction. I thought about my inclination to become addicted to things that make me feel good. Decision time. Regretfully, I tossed the lovely white powder down the toilet, flushed, and never used cocaine again.

While social rules were being redefined in response to the new advocacy movements, another revolution was about to occur that would seriously influence the way ordinary people lived. In 1960, the Federal Drug Administration approved the first oral contraceptive. By the end of that year, "the pill" was being marketed and the sexual revolution had quietly begun.

One outgrowth of the burgeoning interest in sexual innovation was an organization called the Sexual Freedom League. I first heard about it from a psychologist friend who'd been to several of their events in Berkeley, where its activities were flourishing. Up for adventure and fascinated by my friend's lurid tales, I asked him to arrange for me to go to an SFL "party." Amused, he agreed to do so.

Attendance was strictly by referral from someone already in the SFL network. The only other requirement was that everyone had to arrive with a partner of the opposite sex. My friend arranged an escort, a pleasant young man whom I met at dinner, just before we headed out to make our entrance at the sex party as a couple.

On arrival at the apartment where the SFL was meeting, we were each handed a brown paper bag, instructed to write our name on it, remove all our clothes, and place them in the bag. I felt hesitant, suddenly shy, wondering why I was doing this crazy thing. I looked around the living room of the apartment. About fifty people stood about, talking and drinking, looking like any congenial group anywhere, except they were all stark naked.

Slowly I removed my clothes, folding them neatly as if doing so brought some kind of order to what I was about to do. People were drifting into the bedrooms, and after drinking several glasses of wine, I joined the migration. There were three bedrooms. I chose the middle one. As I stood in the doorway, I had to catch my breath I was so shocked at the sight before me. The room was without furniture, the floor a wall-to-wall carpet of bodies in motion. Through the semidarkness it was impossible to see who was doing what to whom, but they all seemed connected in one large undulating mass. There were sounds of moaning and heavy breathing punctuated by short spasmodic screams. I felt immobilized, but I told myself I couldn't just stand in the doorway. I took a deep breath and plunged in, literally.

For the next two hours I melded into the "carpet." One person blurred into the next. I have no idea what was done to me or what I did to anyone else because I felt as though I were in a dream. Whatever I experienced, the feeling was quickly replaced by the distraction of someone new touching me.

On two occasions I did "wake up" enough to become startlingly aware of what was happening. The first time, a man next to me reached over and began to caress the back of another man. Suddenly, all of the action around me stopped. Three people sat straight up.

"We don't do that here," one said. The man withdrew his hand and the action resumed.

So this was strictly heterosexual. No, not quite. The second time I woke up was when someone took my hand and placed it in a hand that was distinctly female. She held tight. I could not see her face since she was one body away, but the female hand began to stroke my palm. It was quite pleasurable, and I was aware of faces around me smiling, too. Sexuality was apparently okay between two women but absolutely taboo between two men. As I realized what was happening, I felt a surge of anger. Sexual freedom as defined by the Sexual Freedom League meant heterosexual freedom. Homosexuality unwelcome. Women didn't even figure in the equation because what women did wasn't important, it didn't threaten anyone—anyone male, that is.

I withdrew my hand and struggled to my feet. I'd had enough. Something was stirring in me, a kind of rage at rejection that I didn't understand. Although I was still convinced I wasn't homosexual, I was nonetheless very angry about what had just happened. How dare these people set the rules for everybody else? That man wasn't hurting anyone. What he did was his own business and that of the person he touched. They had no right to interfere. This growing anger in me was the first hint, I see now, of something that would later take on a life of its own.

I thought I was finished with the Sexual Freedom League, but not quite. A journalist friend in Los Angeles, Joe, heard I'd gone to an SFL party. He'd been assigned to cover one and asked me if I would accompany him. I was curious to see how SFL Berkeley differed from SFL Los Angeles.

Hawaiian Gardens? I didn't even know where that was. The white picket fence did not bode well. Inside, the house was a miracle of bad taste—velvet furniture, shag rugs, chintz drapes, and flowered wallpaper. About a dozen men and women sat in the living room, fully clothed, making small talk. Apparently nothing had started yet.

Joe and I explored the rest of the house. There was the master bedroom which matched the decor of the living room. Three unoccupied children's rooms were complete with teddy bears, tricycles, flaxen-haired dolls, and framed nursery rhymes on the wall. I shuddered at the thought of having sex in any of these rooms.

As we were touring, two couples came out of the living room, entered one of the children's bedrooms, and closed the door. Several other couples disappeared into another child's room, closing the door behind them. Why would anybody want to have sex in a child's bedroom? Must be something I was missing. Maybe these people had children of their own and were turned on by crossing the line of this taboo in so safe and removed a situation. Maybe I just wouldn't think about it.

Soon all the bedroom doors were closed. We rejoined the living room crowd, which had grown in our absence. Couples soon emerged from behind bedroom doors and were replaced by other couples. This was so tame as to be unnerving. Group sex in Hawaiian Gardens consisted of a sedate procession of couples disappearing behind closed doors to do something very quietly that didn't take long. No brown paper bags full of clothes, no writhing bodies all over the floor, no moans, groans, or screams. It was surreal.

I was soon bored with this chaste scene. Joe talked to a few people and we left, giggling all the way to my house, where we tumbled into bed and had an SFL party of our own that was neither chaste nor boring.

I first met Marvin Liebman in the early 1950s when Luce brought him into my bookstore. They had been friends in New York, and now Marvin was working as a fundraiser for a Jewish organization in Los Angeles. A gay man, his politics were left of liberal. He was a talker and a charmer and attracted interesting, accomplished people like a magnet, most of whom he dragged into my shop. In the postbookstore days, Marvin and I remained friends, then we lost touch for a while when he returned to New York to take a public relations job. That job prompted an incredible turnabout in his politics.

In the early 1960s, I was visiting Marvin in New York. By that time he had his own public relations firm, and I was standing in his waiting room, stunned at what I was seeing, a poster touting Dr. Fred Schwartz, a major conservative anticommunist and hatemonger. I had just cut up my Richfield Oil credit card because that company sponsored Schwartz's television program.

"Darling, how wonderful to see you!" Marvin rushed out to greet me, his usual effusive self.

"Marvin, why do you have Fred Schwartz in your waiting room?" I sternly demanded.

"Oh. Well, he's my client. I promote him."

Further conversation revealed that Marvin had become the darling of the country's leading right-wingers, many of whom were his clients and friends. Conservative Charles Edison (son of Thomas Alva and former governor of New Jersey) was his chief benefactor and mentor. Congressman Walter Judd, an old China hand and staunch anticommunist was Marvin's main supporter in his founding of the Committee of One Million to keep Red China out of the United Nations, an objective that Marvin was later personally credited with achieving for fifteen years. William F. Buckley was Marvin's best friend.

"What happened to you, Marvin?"

"Let's go to lunch, darling. I'll explain everything."

He didn't explain anything. He just said it was only business and he didn't really believe all those nasty things these people did. I told him that regretfully we could no longer be friends.

"Don't be ridiculous, darling. We've been friends all these years. We'll be friends the rest of our lives."

"Then we'll have to talk about this political thing."

"Fine."

I quickly learned that I couldn't begin to prevail in a political discussion with Marvin. I was a mere amateur. He was a consummate political professional—he charmed, cajoled, soothed, and lied. I gave up and agreed to a détente so long as he understood that I didn't approve of what he was doing.

In the summer of 1963 I was invited to present a paper at the Third International Congress of Group Psychotherapy in Milan, Italy. When I told Marvin, he was delighted.

"Fabulous, darling. We'll go to Europe together, play for a few weeks, then you can go off to your conference." That sounded great because I'd never been to Europe and Marvin had been many times. My fantasy about him knowing the languages and the ropes collapsed, however, when on our first night out I asked him what I should order from the French menu. He hesitated, then suggested, "This *pamplemousse demi* sounds good." When the half grapefruit arrived as our dinner I realized that Marvin was no more practiced in French than I was. I took four years of French in high school but was always a terrible language student, and anyway I'd slept through most of Miss Brazelton's classes. It was obvious I would have to summon up what language I could and speak for myself.

The Hotel Majestic in Cannes is a great white whale of an edifice overlooking the boulevard de la Croisette and the Bay of Cannes. It is one of the grande dames of the French Riviera. Marvin and I had a bay-view corner suite with bedrooms on either side of a huge parlor.

By the summer of 1963, Marvin and I had settled one important aspect of our relationship. We had tried from time to time to turn our friendship into a romance, but that didn't work for either one of us. After all we were two gay people, though we were both acting within the accepted homosexual ethic of the time—conceal it, deny it, and work around it. Being gay was certainly not something to incorporate into one's identity, much less to build a life around. In a sense, Marvin and I were each other's psychological "beards."

Our first night in Cannes, Marvin had one of his famous attacks of claustrophobia. It had taken me years to get it through my head that Marvin's

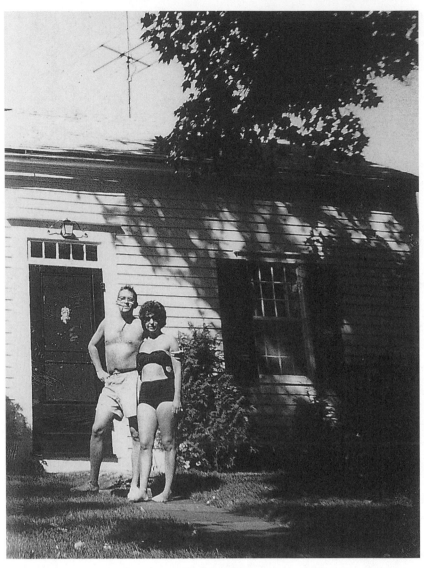

A summer visit with Marvin Liebman at his country house in Connecticut around 1955. We'd been friends since 1952 and would remain friends for the next forty years.

low threshold for boredom was not a reaction to me. I'd seen him fidget and twitch with some of the most fascinating people in the world. This night, lighting one cigarette after another, Marvin paced the floor. Huge billows of smoke collected over his head as he wore a path back and forth across the carpet.

"Good lord, Marvin, what is wrong?"

"Nothing, darling, nothing."

I knew what was wrong, but I decided to ignore it. I went out on our balcony. It was early evening, and the summer air was still and hot. The lights along the Croisette were just flickering on. Bits of French conversation drifted up from the boulevard below amid the hum of traffic and the honking of horns. I felt excited to be where I was, but I knew I had to deal with Marvin sooner or later.

"Okay, Marvin, that's enough. Spit it out!"

Marvin peered at me through the smoke. "Well, here we are. We don't have any plans yet. We don't know anybody yet. I'm restless, that's all." Decoded, he was saying, "Here we are alone with no one to distract us from one another and that is making me nervous."

I reminded him of our New York lunch with his friend Michael Stewart (of "Bye Bye Birdie" fame). Michael had given us a list of friends he had in Cannes, with their phone numbers.

"Call the list," I said.

"I've already called all of them. No one was home."

Sinking into a chair, Marvin looked at me pleadingly.

"Don't you know anyone in Cannes? No, of course you don't. How silly of me."

The fact was I did know someone. José was a ballet dancer whom I'd met through Leslie Carron in the bookstore days, and we'd kept in touch. He'd been with the Paris Ballet but now lived and taught dance in Cannes. I told Marvin.

"Call him, darling, at once!"

José, delighted to hear from me, came over immediately. He was still the beautiful person he'd been when I knew him a decade before—dancer's taut body, cleanly chiseled cheekbones, serious dark eyes, courtly Spanish manner. The three of us piled into our rented car and headed to dinner.

The Colombe d'Or, in St.-Paul-de-Vence, is a magical place. Its walls are hung with paintings by Matisse, Picasso, Chagal, and Miro, all of whom had eaten there in their time. As we walked through the restaurant, an unusual thing happened. Conversation stopped dead and all heads turned toward us. "Look, it's José," I heard someone say in a stage whisper.

When we were seated I asked José what that was all about. He said shyly that he rarely went out in public and people were not used to seeing him. I learned the next day that José was a legend in Cannes because he was a brilliant teacher but so reclusive that a José sighting was something to talk about. I was flattered that this sweet, graceful person came out to do something just for me that he didn't like doing.

Marvin's restlessness had been easily solved that first evening, but it was a different story on many of the nights to follow. As is often the case with some gay men, anonymous sex is the palliative to restlessness. The difference between closeted gay men and closeted lesbians is that gay men always know how to find the sex they need, lesbians don't, or at least I didn't in 1963. Marvin would hit the streets and soon come back with his quarry, hurrying his prize to his own bedroom.

One evening we'd been out to enjoy France's newest form of entertainment—a *discothèque*—where people jammed onto a postage-stamp dance floor and moved to thunderous recorded music. Bodies banged against one another under circling colored lights. We'd finally connected with Michael Stewart's list, and we were having a wonderful time with these New Yorkers transplanted to the French Riviera. The fun of the evening faded, however, when Marvin and I returned to our suite and he immediately began changing his clothes to go out. Suddenly, unexpectedly, I was furious.

"I'm sick of being abandoned every night, Marvin! Why do you get to go out and have these experiences and I'm stuck here?"

"Well, for heaven's sake, darling, let's go and find you a woman!"

I was horrified. At first I wanted to protest that I didn't sleep with women, but Marvin knew that wasn't true, for he had been the person who brokered most of my New York lesbian escapades. "Okay, Marvin, just how do I 'find a woman'?"

"They're all over the place, on the backstreets, standing on the sidewalk."

"A prostitute? You want me to pick up a prostitute?"

"Why not? Come on," and he dragged me out the door before I could think of anything else to say.

As we cruised the dimly lit, narrow streets, Marvin would stop the car each time we saw a woman leaning against a building or standing at the curb alone.

"This one?" he'd ask.

"No," I'd say hurriedly, staring straight ahead. After several of these stops my head began pounding. Was I actually cruising the backstreets of the French Riviera looking for a woman to have sex with? I could feel the panic rising in me. How did I get into this crazy situation? Marvin made me do it. What was I doing with this maniac? He doesn't understand me at all.

"Why are you doing this to me?" I shouted as I began to cry.

"Doing what? I'm only trying to help you."

Marvin stopped the car and I immediately began beating on him with my fists. "Get me out of here, now!" I screamed.

Marvin tried to start the car. In addition to being one of the worst drivers on the planet even in the best of times, he was thoroughly unnerved by my hysterics. He pushed and pulled on the gear shift, metal grinding, the car jerking, lurching like a bucking bronco. Somehow he finally got it to go in the direction of the hotel.

The next morning, lying on the gleaming white sand of the *plage*, I apologized.

"Never mind, darling," he said. "This gay thing is awful, but I'm afraid we're stuck with it." But I didn't believe that for one minute. I agreed that it was awful to be gay, but I certainly wasn't stuck with it.

One day, Marvin went out alone. When he came back, he had a big, blond boy with him. "This is Leon," Marvin said, pushing the boy toward me. Leon flashed a toothy smile and held out his hand.

"Hi, Leon," I said. Leon bowed awkwardly and said, "*Bon jour.*"

"He doesn't speak English," Marvin said.

"And just who or what is Leon and how old is he?" I asked.

"He's a fisherman. I met him down by the docks. He's eighteen."

I took a good look at Leon. Though his shoulders were broad and muscular, his hands were soft and clean. Leon was about as much a fisherman as I was.

"And what are we going to do with Leon?" I asked.

"He's going to be our guide in Cannes."

"But he doesn't speak English."

"We'll manage," said Marvin.

Leon, understanding we were talking about him, flashed his toothy smile again. He was quite handsome, in a pretty-boy way. After that, he was with us constantly. Toward the end of our stay in Cannes, Marvin made the incredible decision to bring Leon back to New York.

"What for?" I foolishly asked.

"Well, darling, to educate and teach him English, of course," Marvin said, a ridiculous smile playing across his face. "I think you're mad," I said. "Doesn't he have a family here?"

"I've already spoken to his father through an interpreter. He's delighted to have his son sponsored for a trip to the States."

"My god, Marvin, you're serious."

"Of course I am, darling. There's just one problem. Because he's of a tender age, I have to apply to the mayor of Cannes for a permit to take him out of France."

"Why is that a problem?"

"Because the mayor is a communist. I have to go to a communist and ask for a favor."

There was a delicious irony in that. Marvin Liebman, the professional anticommunist, going hat in hand to seek approval from a communist, but Marvin did just that. He worked his charm on the mayor and won the okay to have Leon shipped to New York.

The next day Marvin and I left for Paris. He had made all the arrangements and given instructions to Leon's family to send him on the airplane to New York as soon as all his papers were in order. After a few days, Marvin and I parted ways. He returned to New York while I continued touring Europe on my own. I had ten days before my conference was to start.

In London, I met with staff members of the Tavistock Institute to exchange information about our research on groups. In Venice I sat in the sun on the Piazza San Marco and was pinched on the rear by the gondolier as I alighted from his boat. In Florence I visited museums and marveled at the magnificent art and architecture that were everywhere. Finally in Rome, I was ensconced in the Cavalieri Hilton on a hilltop overlooking the gleaming rooftops of the city.

I felt adventurous heading out for a visit to the Trevi Fountain. I threw my coins into the cascading waters, assuring, according to legend, that I would return to Rome. Suddenly I felt the presence of someone standing just behind me.

"Is this your first trip to the Trevi?"

A good-looking, beefy young Italian man was smiling at me.

"Yes, I just arrived in Rome today."

"Hello, my name is Mario. I have lived in your country, Brooklyn. I sold used cars there." Big smile.

We talked and he invited me to dinner. He was polite and friendly, so I saw no harm in accepting. We walked to a restaurant, where over dinner he told me about his Sicilian family and his life in Rome—still selling used cars. He asked me nothing about myself. Coffee arrived and with it Mario's pitch: "Now we will go to my place and make love."

I looked disbelievingly at him.

"I have bought you dinner. I am very nice to you. Now you must be nice to me."

"Not that way, Mario. I hardly know you." I looked around for the door.

"Listen, I know about American girls. I know how to be gentle. You won't be sorry."

I was already sorry. "I think I should go now."

Mario's eyes flashed Sicilian anger. "Bitch!" He reached across the table and slapped me in the face. I was so shocked I couldn't move. He slapped again. That did it. I ran for the door, Mario came right behind me, into the street. I made it to the intersection where a taxi pulled up in response to my frantic waving. I jumped in and fell back against the seat as the cab pulled away. I could see Mario on the curb shaking his fist at me, mouthing curses, his face twisted in anger. I was trembling so I could hardly get the name of the hotel out as I watched the receding figure of my Sicilian suitor through the rear window of the cab. How could I have done such a stupid thing?

Once inside the brightly lit lobby of the Cavalieri Hilton I feel safe in familiar territory, people all around. I breathe easy and make my way to the elevators. No, I could use a drink. I head for the bar off the lobby. Perched on a stool, I think about what just happened to me—comic opera, Italian style, complete with name-calling, face-slapping, and being chased through the streets. I am giggling to myself when I realize suddenly that I am being watched. A man several seats down the bar is staring intently at me. When I look at him, he smiles. Oh no, not again, I think, and I become very busy with my drink.

"Excuse me," he begins, moving to the seat next to mine. "I hope you will not take offense, but I would be very pleased if you would allow me to buy you a drink."

I pause for a moment before turning to him. What could happen to me here in my own hotel?

"Please, may I introduce myself?" he says in a cultured English voice.

"My name is Abdul. I am a guest here in the hotel as I assume you are."
He has a gentleman's bearing, is courteous and well dressed, a far cry from
my Sicilian companion of earlier in the evening.

"Yes, I am staying here."

"Please, if you don't mind my saying so, you looked troubled when you
first came into the bar. Is everything all right?"

I am impressed by the concern in his voice. "Yes, everything is all right,
now," and to my surprise I proceed to tell him all about my adventure with
Mario. He listens very carefully, his face registering sympathy.

"What a terrible experience. I'm so glad you got away from that man.
You're safe now in your own hotel. No harm will come to you here."

Soon, Abdul is telling me his own story. He is a director of the Central
Bank of Iraq, educated in England and in the United States. His parents
died some years before and he had become father to his three younger brothers, who were out of college and married, freeing him to pursue his own
life. He wants to marry and have a family of his own. He pauses, as though
a little embarrassed at having said so much. "But I am too personal perhaps.
Please, tell me about you."

Abdul looks intently interested as I speak. I like that. I like him, and when
he asks if I'd like to go dancing at Le Pergola, the Hilton's roof-garden club,
I accept. Why not? I'm safe here.

The Cavalieri Hilton perches atop the Monte Mario Hill overlooking
Rome. It is somewhat inconveniently located with respect to the center of
the city, but shuttle buses run every hour to the Via Veneto and the Piazza
di Spagna. The inconvenience is compensated for by the spectacular view
of Rome the hotel offers, and nowhere is that view more stunning than from
Le Pergola.

Abdul and I dance for hours and I hardly notice the effects of the Strega
that has succeeded my gin and tonic in a bow to Italian custom. "It is the
most Italian of drinks, so delicious and mellow. You must try it," Abdul
insists. It is delicious, and I am soon quite mellow. We close Le Pergola and
before I realize what is happening I am in Abdul's room, but I don't care.
I realize how lonely I have been since Marvin's departure. I'm glad to have
Abdul's companionship and he seems glad to have mine, that night and the
next day and night, and the next, three days of sipping Strega and feeling
mellow enough to agree to almost anything Abdul wants to do. We shop
on the Via Veneto, sightsee, and spend long hours in the sun at the Cavalieri
Hilton's beautiful pool.

On the third day of our "romance," Abdul becomes very serious. He says he has something important to talk to me about. He begins by telling me that all of his brothers have American wives and that he, too, desires to be married to an American. He says he thinks we could have a wonderful life together. He asks me to marry him.

I am so astonished I don't know what to say. I have grown fond of Abdul, but after two days and three nights he is still a virtual stranger. I've had no thoughts of an actual relationship with him. This is summer in Rome, a time out, not real life, but Abdul knows what he wants and he pursues it.

When I find my voice, I say weakly, "Abdul, I can't marry you. I'm Jewish. Where would we live? I can't live in an Arab country."

"Oh no no, that's not a problem," he hastily reassures me. "We will live in Beirut. It's a beautiful modern city, very sophisticated and liberal-minded. It's the Paris of the Middle East. You'll love it there."

I tell Abdul I will think about it. Actually, I'm struck by the irony of the situation. I do want to get married, but everything about this proposal is wrong—wrong culture, wrong continent, wrong script all together. I'm grateful that I'm leaving for Milan the next day. That night I gently tell Abdul that I cannot accept his offer of marriage. He is very disappointed as he writes out his address in Iraq and asks me to please contact him if I change my mind. I say I will and that I've had a wonderful three days with him, which I would never forget. I was right about that part, but for reasons I had no hint of at the time.

Arriving in Milan, I was quickly drawn into the Third International Congress of Group Psychotherapy. Given that it was the 1960s, it didn't seem particularly bizarre that a Dutch psychologist presented on a therapy group in which all the members took LSD at each session, including him, for he wanted to be on the same "psychological plane" as his patients. Another presentation was on a therapy group designed to "cure" homosexuality. The group was made up of male homosexuals and beautiful girls. The results were termed "inconclusive." As for me, I made my presentation, saw old friends, and made new ones.

The hottest gossip of the Congress revolved around what appeared to be the galloping senility of the elderly president of the International Council of Group Psychotherapy, Dr. J. L. Moreno, well-known for his invention of "psychodrama." In most of his presentations Dr. Moreno made no sense at all. The delegates were already short-tempered because of the suffocating heat in the unairconditioned palace of the Provincial Government of Milan where the conference was held. Frustration and heat exhaustion finally combined to cause the audience to abandon civility and boo the famous Dr. Moreno off the stage.

J. L.'s wife, Zerka, was everywhere at this conference trying to take over for her failing husband but audiences were no kinder to this aggressive lady, distinctive in appearance because she had only one arm. Compassion for the Morenos gave way to annoyance with them. I was appalled at the behavior of the grownup professional attendees and I hoped that when my turn came to lose my mental compass, I would have the sense to stay home. I felt sorry for Zerka but this was not to be my last encounter with her.

Several years after the Milan meetings, I visited the Moreno Institute in Manhattan to observe a demonstration of psychodrama techniques. Zerka was the demonstrator. She asked for volunteers to join her on the stage. No one came forward. She entreated and cajoled. Nothing. Exasperated, she came down into the audience, grabbed my arm, and led me up the stairs onto the stage. I didn't like it, but I went along.

Zerka sat opposite me and began asking questions. I told her who I was and why I was in New York. She then leaned forward and looked into my eyes. I felt a chill go down my spine. She was moving in for the kill, setting me up for a conflict that could be played out in the psycho-drama mode. I felt tense and I reminded myself that I didn't have to tell her anything. I was shifting uncomfortably in my chair when she asked her question, slowly and deliberately. "Who did you have breakfast with this morning?"

I sat very still. How could she know to ask that? Did she just look at me and see "queer"? Something inside me tipped. I had just come away from one of my lesbian adventures, and I wanted to shout back at her, "Okay, I slept with a woman last night. So what? Who cares?" but I actually said, "It's none of your business!"

Zerka smiled. She had me. After that I could hear Zerka's voice, but my mind wandered away. Why was I so panicked by this exchange? Zerka didn't matter. She couldn't hurt me. It was I who made judgments about homosex-uality. I was the one who condemned myself for being attracted to women. I was the one to watch out for.

Suddenly, I knew I had to get out of there, away from Zerka, that audience, my own thoughts, but I felt leaden, unable to rise. With all my strength I forced my body out of the chair. Unsteadily, I descended the few stairs from the stage. Eyes straight ahead, I walked up the aisle to the back of the auditorium. The audience watched in silence. Zerka said nothing. Out on the street, I hurried into the New York night, away from unnerving questions, prying eyes, and coming too close to losing control of my secret.

❦ 11

Back in La Jolla, the doctor broke the news to me gently. I was pregnant. There was no doubt who the father was because Abdul was the only man I'd had sex with in recent months. Mellowed out on Strega during my three days in Rome, I had ignored such practical considerations as preventing pregnancy. Now that lapse in judgment became a major crisis in my life.

Should I have the baby? I knew myself well enough to answer the question honestly. I was very involved in my work and the idea of committing at this point in my life to the kind of time a child needs and deserves felt overwhelming. I couldn't even imagine coping with a pregnancy. I didn't want to be unfair to an innocent child. I had been born to not-ready-for-parenthood teenagers whose mixed feelings about parental responsibilities played out in a way that created lifelong emotional problems for me. I didn't want to do that to someone else. I decided I would have an abortion.

Abortion in 1963 was a dicey proposition. I'd heard hair-raising tales about women being mutilated or bleeding to death in back-alley operations that terrified me. Abortion was a crime, I could even be arrested. It was too frightening to think about, but one thing was clear. I had to make this decision quickly. No time to sit around obsessing, so not quite knowing what I was doing, I began the search.

Following a trail of referrals, I talked to people all over the country, collecting names and phone numbers and horror stories. Ultimately, the referral that sounded the safest and easiest was practically right next door, in Tijuana. I discovered that the abortion clinics there were run by qualified medical doctors and functioned semi-openly—no cloak-and-dagger intrigue, no switching cars in deserted parking lots, no traveling blindfolded so you wouldn't know where you had been.

I was advised not to mention the word "abortion" in my initial phone call but to simply say I was calling for an "appointment." My instructions from the Tijuana clinic were to fast for eight hours before my "appointment" and to bring $350 in cash. I was relieved to hear that I would have a local anesthetic and could return to San Diego the same night. My dear friends, Bob and Dorothy Gray, agreed to accompany me, for which I was thankful. Although I was in good hands, I still felt scared to death.

When we arrived at the clinic, we were ushered into a small office. The doctor was waiting for us. He was a neat little man in a clean white coat who asked me questions about my general health then explained what he was going to do and how long it would take. He was gentle and kind, and when he asked for the $350, I was only too glad to hand it over. Instructing the Grays to remain in his office, he led me down the hall to the operating room.

I was laid out on an operating table attended by four uniformed nurses. The room was well lit and clean. The procedure took about twenty minutes. I didn't feel anything. Then I was taken to a recovery room where I fell asleep, feeling quite relaxed and thankful that it was over. As I slept, the Grays waited in the doctor's office. Bob Gray, being a curious soul, decided to investigate the closet behind the doctor's desk. He cautiously opened the door to find the closet piled high with suitcases. Were they full of money, or clothes for a quick getaway, or both? His curiosity did not extend to examining the contents of the luggage, fortunately, because at that moment the doctor returned to his office. Bob was back in his chair as the door opened.

I was given a sheet of paper as we left the clinic, the "postoperative instructions," including how to reach the doctor if I had any questions. Several phone numbers were listed for him, demonstrating how open that clinic was.

The Grays and I drove back to La Jolla, where I had arranged to see my own doctor. In an act of kindness I will never forget, he met me in his office on a Friday night to check me out and make sure I was okay. His kindness was underlined by the fact that he was Catholic, had nine kids, and was not exactly a fan of abortion. I realized even then that I was extremely lucky to have had such a benign experience, so unlike what happened to many women, botched, butchered, infected, or terrorized by the threat of being caught.

The following year there was an election in Tijuana and the city was "cleaned up." All the abortion clinics moved to Juarez, where they operated until January 22, 1973, when the U.S. Supreme Court declared American anti-abortion laws unconstitutional. That decision eliminated the need for trips to Mexico or hazardous ventures into the world of back-alley abortion mills where being maimed or killed was always a possibility. Now, more than three decades later, it is grotesque to think that a repressive political climate might someday bring back the nightmare of illegal abortions, that women might once again have to risk death to implement the choice that should be theirs alone. Only in a country where laws are made mostly by men would such a calamity even be thinkable. In the meantime, legal abortion puts at risk only the courageous doctors and nurses whose own lives are on the line from the guns and bombs of lunatics on the religious right.

I was asked recently by someone who knew I'd had an abortion if I ever regretted it. Did I ever think about "Little Abdul" who would, at this writing, be thirty-eight years old? Yes, I have thought about that and about the delights and the difficulties having such a son would have brought. And then there would be the child himself. He would, no doubt, be interested in knowing his father, as he would have a right to do. Assuming Abdul, Sr., was still living in Iraq, there would be that country's anti-Americanism and anti-Semitism to deal with, or we might even be at war with Iraq.

But why make it so complicated when it was so simple? I made a decision that was right for my life in 1963. I do not regret it, not for a minute.

Michael Murphy bore a startling resemblance to the movie star Tyrone Power. His long, dark eyelashes shadowed a face that was boyishly handsome and innocently seductive, almost angelic. He was kidlike in his enthusiasm for the project he was just getting underway.

My involvement in the Human Potential Movement began in January 1964, when I attended an invitational weekend seminar at Big Sur Hot Springs to hear its proprietor talk about his plans for a unique seminar center to be developed on his family-owned 150-acre site overlooking the Pacific Ocean. Little did Michael, or any of us, know that we were about to launch an international movement, reordering values and behavior for hundreds of thousands of people who would attend his seminars or those at the many growth centers around the world that would spin off his. The Esalen Institute was born that weekend.

My introduction to Big Sur Hot Springs was unnerving. It began with my arrival at the Monterey Airport where I was met by a long-haired, bearded mountain man who grunted that he was from the "Springs" and told me to go sit in his truck while he collected my luggage. Soon we were off, lurching over the Big Sur road with such a clattering of metal parts that I feared the ancient vehicle would fly apart before we ever got to the "Springs."

Conversation in that truck was impossible, which was fine with me because I needed to concentrate on willing this vehicle to stay on the road on the hairpin turns, for which the driver neither slowed nor braked. I told myself that he probably drove this route all the time, and he was still in one piece, a thought that allowed me to relax just enough to take in the breathtaking sight that is the Big Sur coastline.

The wild ride ended in front of the Hot Springs Lodge, where the truck screeched to a halt and the driver, dumping my bags, mumbled something I didn't understand and roared off in a cloud of dust. Looking around, the first thing I saw was the sparkling Pacific Ocean at the base of the cliff, calm and peaceful, the sunlight bouncing off its surface. Then I saw the buildings that made up the Hot Springs compound, charming, quaint structures, some of which looked like they might blow over in a strong wind. I registered inside the lodge and was shown to my cabin. As I examined the little building that was to be my home for the next few days, I asked myself why I had decided to attend this weekend since country living was not exactly something I was drawn to.

The cabin had a door that didn't quite close and a window that obviously hadn't been opened in years. The creaking wooden floor supported a bed and a chair. That was it. A rod suspended between two posts served as the closet. I was inspecting the minuscule bathroom when I heard a scraping sound behind me. I turned to face a small furry animal poised in the open doorway. Our eyes met. Because I had no idea what this thing was or what it had a mind to do, I stood perfectly still. After a minute or so, my furry friend, his inspection completed, turned and skittered away. I slammed the door, which bounced back open again.

The dining room of the Hot Springs Lodge was as rough-hewn as the rest of the place, but its candle-lit interior had a warm, cozy feeling about it. It was there that the first meeting of the weekend was held with the forty invited guests, most of whom would eventually become the Who's Who of the Human Potential Movement. The weekend also featured lectures and demonstrations. Bernie Gunther previewed the techniques that would make him the massage guru of the 1960s. Tony Sutich was a psychologist who was completely paralyzed from the neck down. He spoke about future plans for the *Journal of Humanistic Psychology*, of which he was the founder and editor.

Flat on his back on a gurney, this extraordinary man was unable to move anything but his mouth and eyes. Virginia Satir told her ideas for doing therapy with families, work for which she would later become celebrated around the world.

When the meeting was over we were all led along a moon-lit path down to "the baths," a spectacular arrangement of large wooden tubs set into the side of the cliff and open to the sea. Shedding our clothes, we sank into the warm mineral waters flowing into the tubs from the hot springs. With the chill ocean air on my face and the warm swirling waters caressing my body, I wanted to stay right where I was forever. The Esalen tubs became famous for their soothing effect, and for a few other kinds of experiences that were rumored to be often available under the dark surface of those swirling waters.

It was a spectacular weekend, and I was hooked on the astonishing beauty of the Hot Springs with its miniature rain forests, rolling hills, and lush green fields dotted by vegetable gardens and colorful flower beds. The ocean could be seen from everywhere on the property, offering a dramatic backdrop to all things exotic that Esalen would come to stand for.

In 1964 I conducted my first workshop at Esalen. It was designed to help people stop smoking, but the "stop smoking" groups were soon replaced by a workshop that grew out of a personal dilemma of my own. It started like this. One day I was talking to a psychologist friend, Tom. I was bemoaning my inability to find the proper mate, which I attributed to the dearth of marriageable men in La Jolla. I'd dated most of the bachelors around, and I'd either found some terrible flaw in each one or just let the relationship slip away for no discernable reason. Tom asked if I met men in the workshops I did. I said I hadn't thought of workshops as a spousal hunting ground because I felt ethically bound not to become involved with clients.

"Bullshit," Tom said. "Leading workshops is not therapy. It's a time-limited contact. You don't have an ongoing relationship with these people. Most of them come to workshops in the first place looking for love. Design a workshop for single people, then you, my dear, can have the pick of the litter."

The more I thought about it, the more I liked the idea. No one was doing such a group. It could help people explore the truth about how they went about looking for love. The Quest for Love workshop was an instant hit. Wherever I did it, people signed up in large numbers. I became a growth center "circuit rider," doing the Quest for Love in cities along the East Coast, in the deep South, in the Midwest, up and down California. It was fascinating to compare how people participated in different regions of the country. The easterners were talky, intellectual, and combative. The southerners were courteous and aloof, always mindful of protocol. The midwesterners were uptight and slow to move toward one another. The Californians fell into each other's arms, eager to demonstrate how uninhibited they were.

But what of my own quest for love? The prize continued to elude me. Again and again, I was attracted to a man, dated, hoped, lost interest, and moved on. In one instance, I did not move on, but by design the relationship did not move on either.

When I met Esalen's Mike Murphy, he was in his early thirties, unmarried, and monastically celibate, just out of an ashram. On a trip to San Francisco we went out one evening. After dinner he said he'd like to do something he'd never done. He wanted to go to a porno movie. I was amused and delighted to accompany him on this maiden voyage. I had seen sexually explicit films before, so I felt like an old pro.

We had fun, giggling to cover up our embarrassment at what was happening on the screen and in the theater, but this experience seemed to sexualize things between us. We began a dalliance that went on for several years with the tacit understanding that neither of us was going to take it too seriously— a friendship with a sexual component. Both of us were traveling a lot in those days, and we often found ourselves in the same city. By then we were keeping count of the cities we'd dallied in.

One trip was particularly memorable because during it our determination to defy emotional involvement was tested. It was a hot, sticky summer in New York. We were invited to dinner at Bill Schutz's. Bill was a social psychologist who would later move to Esalen, become a major star in the Human Potential Movement, and rise to fame on late-night television talk shows for having people fall backwards into his arms to demonstrate how interpersonal trust works. I liked Bill and his then-wife, Liz, who at the time of our visit was in her eighth or ninth month of pregnancy. Quite generous of her to be cooking dinner for us, I thought.

The trouble with Michael began in the taxi on the way to Bill's apartment. He was talking avidly about something, waving his hands around, his face animated, his eyes shining with excitement. I stared at him, so handsome, so dear, so smart, and suddenly I felt a stirring within me of feelings I'd never had before—I was in love with him. I wanted to interrupt him to say what I was feeling, but I was acutely aware that this feeling was against the rules of our relationship. I knew I should keep it to myself, but in the elevator I just blurted it out. "Michael, I think I'm in love with you."

He looked very alarmed. "Well, you know, uh," he stammered, "you know how I feel about you, but we just have fun together. That's what we decided, isn't it?"

We'd reached Bill's floor. Having buzzed us in, Bill was standing in the hallway to greet us. I felt stupid for starting that conversation in the elevator. At dinner Michael was his usual effervescent self. The conversation centered on Human Potential Movement gossip. I had the strangest feeling that maybe the conversation in the elevator hadn't really happened. Then, after dinner, Bill suggested that we go out somewhere. I had purposely worn my basic black dress and pearls for just this suggestion. I loved going out in New York.

"I have a special place I'd like to take you," Bill said. Then he looked at what Michael was wearing and said, "I don't think those clothes will do." Michael looked quite well dressed to me, but Bill disappeared into the bedroom and returned with a pair of khaki shorts, similar to the ones he was wearing. He insisted Michael put them on even though they were about three sizes too big. Michael looked ridiculous.

"Bill, just where is it we're going?" I inquired.

"You'll see," he said.

The four of us piled into Bill's Porsche convertible and pulled into Manhattan traffic. Not far away we stopped in front of a seedy, run-down hotel. What in the world were we going to do? See porno films? Why did Michael have to wear khaki shorts? *Make* porno films?

Liz and I followed Bill and Michael into a huge brightly lit basement room that was very hot and reeked of disinfectant. Though my interest was piqued, I was beginning to feel annoyed. Then I saw the Ping-Pong tables, row upon row of them, a table tennis club, we were in a Ping-Pong club! Bill motioned Liz and me to sit down as he disappeared and returned with two paddles and some Ping-Pong balls. I couldn't believe this was happening—Bill and Michael were going to play Ping-Pong while Liz and I sat and watched! This was an evening out in New York? Michael looked delighted. Liz looked tranquil, but then she caught me looking at her and confessed, "Bill loves to play Ping-Pong. What can I tell you?"

By then I was seething. How dare these people just assume I was satisfied to passively sit and watch Ping-Pong? I didn't sign up to be anybody's "little woman." I was furious at Michael, too. Suddenly he was not a grown man at all, but a little boy in those ridiculous shorts, blameless, innocent, a child without guile. What did that make me? Stupid, romantic, in love with love, out of touch?

I didn't express my anger that night. I felt at a loss to know what to do, so I did nothing, swallowed my pride and my anger, wondering if there was something essential about relationships between men and women that I just didn't get. Whatever feelings about Michael I'd had earlier in the evening were gone. I believe he sensed this and was relieved. We were just pals again, babes in toyland, sexual buddies, making no demands on one another's lives. It was the 1960s, everything changing, new rules, new roles, life and love not what they used to be, not yet what they were going to become.

When I think back to the work we did in the Human Potential Movement in the 1960s I am struck by the far-reaching effects our programs have had. Small groups are routinely used now, nearly forty years later, in a great variety of settings to open up communication, teach interpersonal skills, improve organizational functioning, enable deeper, more satisfying relationships, and give comfort to people dealing with life-altering problems.

The question we should perhaps have asked ourselves more often in those days of intensive encounter was whether people changed by their experiences with us where it really counted, in their everyday lives. In our workshops we were terribly invested in dramatic demonstrations of our ability to penetrate defenses, rip away the veils, and get to the authentic person. I wonder now if we didn't frequently neglect the next step, helping individuals integrate new insights and behaviors so that they could fit them into the repertoire of their real lives.

I know that some people left our workshops feeling reborn, newly in touch with their potential for loving and experiencing, ready for a more exciting trip, only to find the people at home still doing business at the same old stand—bored, complaining, stuck in routines, and afraid to try anything new. Our participants came back with such stories, and back, and back, bringing significant others with them, friends, family, even neighbors, until they could begin to feel a community of intimates around them. If we did anything for these folks it was to create an ethic of responsibility for changing the ambience of their life, working on attachments that were authentic and deeply felt, and getting rid of shallow and toxic relationships. This was a kind of activism of the soul, pushing for change at the most personal level possible. I liked being an agent of change. It made me feel worthwhile and affecting.

An important development for me in the Human Potential Movement of the 1960s was the opening of a new growth center right in my backyard. Eventually there would be over a hundred of these centers throughout the United States and around the world. The first was Esalen, the second was Kairos. Just outside San Diego in a lovely country setting, Kairos was the brainchild of Bob and Patti Driver, a vibrant young couple every bit as idealistic as Michael Murphy, but where Michael was the slim, dark, ascetic, Bob Driver was a Norse warrior, tall and sturdy, with a mass of curly reddish hair, piercing blue eyes, and a great ruddy beard. His enthusiasm for life was infectious. Being around Bob, Patti, and their five children was a warm and loving experience. I did so many workshops at Kairos that it became my second home.

A few years later, when I moved back to Los Angeles from San Diego, I opened one of the first urban growth centers, Kairos–Los Angeles. It was during this time of working with the Drivers that Bob first became ill with the leukemia that would take his life at thirty-four. Watching this robust young man fall ill, come back energetically, slide again into exhaustion, become frail and finally succumb to the disease was an overwhelming experience for me. I had never watched anyone die before. I felt so powerless, so outraged at the injustice of it.

I often wonder what it would be like to know the future before it happens. Would it soften the blows, or make life too terrifying to be able to go on? A few years after Bob's death, I watched my dear friend Roberto die of cancer at thirty-three and felt the same sadness and outrage. And several decades later I would witness the deaths of many friends, clients, and colleagues from AIDS. The sadness and outrage, multiplied by the thousands, became numbing, one of the mind's devices for preserving sanity.

CRXD 12

It is early January, 1968. I am forty years old today. There are certain birthdays that are veiled warnings of danger—new challenges, loss of comfort, threat of the unknown.

Forty is one of those birthdays, the signal year in which one's life comes under attack from within. Am I where I planned to be? Am I who I wanted to be? Am I doing what I should be doing?

I am acutely aware that I am alone, glancing frequently through the expansive glass walls of my La Jolla house to catch a visitor approaching even though I know there will be no visitors because I have invited none. I eat dinner from a tray in front of the television. I try not to think about why I have done this weird thing of shutting everyone out of my birthday. It makes no sense because in my isolation I feel angry and abandoned. Where is everybody?

I kept telling myself that I should plan something for my birthday, that's what people do, but now Saturday has come and I am alone. I busy myself with household tasks, cleaning closets, reorganizing drawers. I am bringing order to an already orderly household, but doing this gives me a feeling that everything is as it should be.

This birthday is a special one. Maybe I'm trying to avoid the specialness of it. My mind goes back to my sixteenth, another special birthday. My mother bought a cake and we waited for my father to come home to celebrate. He never came, apparently forgetting that it was my birthday. My mother went to bed crying, her usual solution to my father's transgressions. Alone, I sang happy birthday to myself and dumped the cake in the trash. I was beyond tears, hardening my resolve to never again expect anything to work out for me in this failed family. Was I replicating my miserable sixteenth now on my lonely fortieth? I don't sing happy birthday to myself. I just go to bed early.

I have the dream that night, the one I've had before. In the dream, I return to my house, but there are other people living there. They open the door but look right through me. I am invisible. The door shuts in my face. I want to cry, but I can't. I run away. I wander the streets. I must find a place to stay. I go into hotels. I go from room to room, but none is satisfactory, and I leave in frustration. Then I see a house where a party is going on. It's my house again. I go in. Everyone is having a wonderful time, laughing, dancing, talking. Some of the people look familiar to me. I know them from somewhere. I'm eager to say hello, but when I approach them they quickly turn away from me. I feel devastated. Where do I belong? I cannot find a place to be. Suddenly I am back in the streets, panicky, unable to get my bearings. I ask passersby where I am, but they rush away without answering. I look up at tall buildings and feel very small and helpless, a child, frightened and alone.

Sunday morning I awaken with a start. I feel strangely detached, not sure where I am. The mood of the dream is still with me. I get up and pass myself in the mirror. The person I see there looks ravaged. She glares back at me, eyes half-closed, face drawn by fatigue. She looks like she's had a hard night. I hear a voice. Where is it coming from? "You are forty years old and something is wrong."

"Something is wrong? What does that mean? My life is great. I do rewarding work, I have a secure job, an active social life, terrific friends."

My mind tries to stay with these thoughts but it keeps slipping back to the dream, to the party where I am not recognized, to the house where I live but I don't. Where do I belong? I go back to bed and let the tears come. I have been so afraid of this. I am in the crisis I have feared, this is why I am alone on this day, to confront the charade, to see that the only way to be free of the burden of my secret is for there to no longer be a secret. I am terrified of this, but on my fortieth birthday I come face to face with myself and I know I must stop the charade. I know I am homosexual. I can no longer hide. I have to do something about it.

I had a feeling of déjà vu about my decision. Once before, at Stanford, I had decided that if I were homosexual I couldn't do it there. Now I seemed faced with the same dilemma—if I'm going to be gay, I can't do it in La Jolla. Were there gay people in La Jolla? I'd never known any. The thought of being a lesbian in La Jolla was horrifying. Actually the thought of being a lesbian anywhere was horrifying. I hated that word. Maybe I could just be gay.

The matter was easily settled. Bell & Howell was publishing my ENCOUNTERTAPES, with elegant packaging and a commercial promotion campaign. I'd been to the company's headquarters in Lincolnwood, Illinois, and met with Pete Peterson, the young CEO and president of Bell & Howell. He liked me and my project, and when I asked for a job, he immediately hired me to work for a Bell & Howell subsidiary, the Atlanta-based Human Development Institute, with my own office in Los Angeles. All I had to do was continue to develop ENCOUNTERTAPE programs. I negotiated not only an office but a secretary and a research assistant.

My transition away from La Jolla stretched through March. There were times when I had doubts about the wisdom of leaving so secure an existence. Some days I would just sit in my office staring at the wall and obsessing: Was I doing something liberating, or was it crazy and self-destructive?

"I'm not sure just what it is that I'm doing," I confided to Sid Jourard, the brilliant psychologist who had written *The Transparent Self*. Sid and I had crossed paths often at conferences and growth centers around the country. He was in town to do a workshop at Kairos and he stopped by to say hello. I was in a funk about the changes I was making, so when Sid asked what was wrong, I told him. He smiled and nodded. "What you're doing is reinventing yourself," he said. His words hit a chord. What a positive way to think about it—I was reinventing myself.

On the day I arrived in Los Angeles to live in 1968, I was scheduled to do a Quest for Love workshop at a local growth center. Miriam, the volunteer coordinator, had efficiently organized the forty participants, and I was grateful to her for everything running so smoothly. I'd spoken to Miriam on the phone, but I'd not yet met her in person, so when she suggested we have dinner after the workshop I readily agreed.

It wasn't until we were in the restaurant that I actually looked at Miriam. She had a bright, open face and crystal-clear blue eyes. She spoke with a vitality that was engaging. Short, with a Rubenesque build, there was a certain sensuousness about her that I felt attracted to immediately, surprising myself. I wasn't accustomed to letting such feelings come through. I had to remind myself that it was okay now. I was allowed. It still made me uncomfortable.

Miriam was about my age, divorced, three adolescent children, enthusiastically involved in her work as a growth center volunteer. Miriam was a talker and I liked listening to her animated delivery, lots of energy in her voice and her face. I also liked watching her soft body shift as she spoke, as if her enthusiasm exerted such force that she couldn't sit still.

In the week following my dinner with Miriam I thought about her a lot. I was pleased when she called me to get together again. This time she came to my house. During dinner, my mind kept slipping out of the conversation, like a phonograph needle sliding out of its groove. I thought about how nice it might be to hold that soft body. I wondered what it would be like to kiss her mouth? Then I would shake myself awake. My god, this woman wasn't even gay as far as I knew. What was I thinking? Immediately, my censor went to work: Miriam was a San Fernando Valley housewife. She liked me, she was nice to me. Am I going to fall in love with every woman who is nice to me? I had no reference point for this. I'd fallen into my relationship with Luce, no courtship, no pursuit. It just happened. I realized I hadn't the vaguest idea how to court a woman. I felt stupid, then Miriam interrupted my reverie.

"Hello? Are you there? You seem to have gone away," she said.

I felt embarrassed. "Sorry, just got lost in thought," I stammered.

"Thinking about what?"

"Oh nothing, really."

"I don't believe you."

Miriam looked me straight in the eye. I felt caught and thought about lying, but that didn't feel right. "I was thinking about you."

Miriam smiled. "Good. Because I've been thinking about you."

Could I have heard that right? I searched Miriam's face for a clue as to what she meant. She was staring at me intently. I wanted to look away, but I couldn't. We must have stayed that way, staring at one another, for several minutes. It seemed like an eternity.

I reached across the table and took Miriam's hand. She let me do it. I could feel my heart trying to beat its way out of my chest. Slowly, I stood up and went around the table. I leaned over Miriam and kissed her, a long, lingering kiss. Her mouth tasted sweet. She seemed sure of what she was doing. I wondered . . . then decided not to think at all. We were moving toward the bedroom, still kissing.

The rest of the night was a mixture of incredible tenderness and overwhelming passion. We pressed ourselves together, holding in the ecstasy to feel it, first in one body and then in the other, and then in both at once, losing the boundaries between us, reaching a kind of unity that was beyond understanding or even the desire to understand. I had never experienced so much in so many parts of my body for so long a time. We stopped only when exhaustion demanded it. With the morning light, we slept.

That was the beginning of a year-long relationship in which I was more open than I had ever been to a loving sexual connection with a woman. There was none of the ambivalence I'd felt when I was with Luce. I loved being with Miriam and when we weren't together I missed her terribly. I was so taken with what was happening in our sexual life that I hardly noticed that we didn't have a life outside of bed.

Gradually it became apparent that Miriam was more troubled than I'd suspected about the nature of our relationship. She didn't introduce me to her family or her friends. She was not interested in meeting mine. We fought about her seeming resistance to being integrated into my life in any way, and as her conflict about being involved with a woman came increasingly to the surface, I could no longer hide my awareness of it.

I was perplexed. Miriam claimed she had never before been attracted to a woman as she was to me. I had difficulty believing her, but she stuck to her story. She said over and over that she had simply fallen in love with me, that this experience was about me, not about being gay. She insisted that for her the quality of passion did not feel different being with a man or with a woman. I didn't know what to believe about her. Was Miriam in denial of her sexuality? She was certainly in conflict about what was happening, and that conflict caused her to retreat from me. I had learned so much from this sensual woman about opening up to my own sexuality that the possibility of losing her felt unbearable. I tried once more to bind us together in life.

After much discussion, Miriam finally agreed to bring her sixteen-year-old daughter, Cindy, to my house for dinner. Cindy turned out to be a delightful young woman, clearly wise beyond her years. Miriam fidgeted, nervously talked about nothing in particular, forgot to eat. Finally, Cindy put her fork down and looked affectionately at her mother.

"Listen, Mom, will you settle down? I know that you and Betty are lovers, and I think it's terrific. So relax, will you?"

Miriam gazed in disbelief at her daughter. Cindy reached over and patted her mother's hand.

"Just relax, it's all right."

Miriam's eyes filled with tears. "What a kid," she said, shaking her head, "and what a dope I am."

I was quick to agree with her on both counts.

I'd hoped Cindy's understanding and acceptance would be enough to calm Miriam's inner turmoil, but it wasn't. She withdrew more and more. I felt so empty without her, yearned to have my arms around her, hear her voice. I called her but she didn't want to talk to me. I sat staring at the phone, trying to will her to call me. I ached, was overwhelmed with sadness, and had no idea how I was ever going to get through this.

What I gradually came to realize was how important a transitional relationship my connection with Miriam had been. She was either not ready to be gay, possibly not gay at all, but her gift to me was the opportunity to experience intimacy with a woman without the conflict that I had felt so deeply in the past. I was committed to continuing my search, though where, how, and with whom I couldn't imagine.

Because I was still grieving the loss of my relationship with Miriam, I welcomed the distraction of a multicity tour of the Quest for Love workshop with a dear friend, Fred Stoller. Fred was the innovative psychologist who co-invented marathon groups and developed the use of videotape feedback in encounter groups. A few days before we were scheduled to leave on the tour, I went to my doctor for a routine checkup. He found a small lump in my left breast and insisted I see a surgeon right away. I was dispatched to the office of Dr. K, a breast surgery specialist.

Shortly after I was admitted to Dr. K's office, I had a peculiar feeling—something was not right there. Was I nervous? Yes, but it was more than that. In a cold, precise manner, Dr. K posed his questions: "Do you have any health problems?" "Have you ever had surgery?" "Are your parents alive?" "Are they in good health?" My feeling that something in this office was odd persisted. My eyes wandered from Dr. K's face to the diplomas on the wall, to the pictures of children on the credenza behind him, to his desk.

"Has anyone in your family ever had breast cancer?"

Breast! That was it! Dr. K's desk was shaped like a breast! I took a closer look. The desk was a half-cylinder that came to a point at the front, the nipple aimed right at me. The doctor sat in the hollowed-out space at the back of the breast. My mind began to race. Did Dr. K have a breast-shaped bed, a breast-shaped house? He began to look surreal to me, going in and out of focus, grotesque and menacing behind his breast.

"Excuse me. I have to leave now."

The doctor looked bewildered.

"I just have to leave," I said.

Outside I wondered if I'd been hallucinating. Did he really have a breast-shaped desk? It didn't matter. Real or not, that breast was aimed right at me. Calming myself, I telephoned my internist.

"I need another referral. I can't see Dr. K."

"Why not?"

"Because he has a desk shaped like a breast."

Silence on the other end.

"It's too unnerving, don't you see?"

"You're understandably anxious . . ."

"I need another referral."

"Okay."

Dr. F was a warm, affable fellow who sat behind a normal desk. He recommended immediate surgery to determine whether the lump was malignant. Mammography was not yet in use, so it was necessary to open up and have a look. I told the doctor that I was about to go on tour. Cancel, he advised, but no, too many people were involved. I'd take my chances. Be back in a month. Schedule me then. I felt fine, making it difficult to appreciate the urgency of the situation. I was scared but also excited about the trip. What difference could a few weeks make?

I waited until Fred and I were in the first city to tell him. At dinner one evening, I said, "I think I might have cancer."

Fred put his fork down and looked at me. "What are you doing here? Why aren't you in a hospital?"

"I didn't want to miss the trip."

"My god, aren't you worried?"

"Yes, but I'm going to put it out of my mind."

Fred's eyes filled with tears. "I couldn't stand for something to happen to you. I really care about you."

"Nothing's going to happen to me. C'mon, you and I are tough. We'll be on the road doing workshops together twenty years from now."

But I was wrong. Several months later, Fred was standing in line at a bank when he had a heart attack and died on the spot. He was forty-six years old. My breast lump was benign. I never felt vulnerable with this lump despite knowing that it could have been cancer. Denial is a powerful ally, but denial didn't work with Fred's death. I was shaken and scared by it, by how unpredictable life is, and the irony of it being Fred and not me. It was Fred's death that made me feel fragile, the suddenness of it, no warning. That terrified me.

Early June, 1968. I looked around the rather grim room in the basement of the Glide Memorial Church in San Francisco, where I would spend four days in straight-backed discomfort conducting an Esalen-sponsored Quest for Love workshop for six people. Something was weird here—a small circle of wooden chairs, a cold cavernous room—an Esalen experience should be had in the open air, under sunlit trees, sprawled on the grass, listening to the ocean lapping against the rocks. Why did I ever agree to do this damn workshop?

The people arrived. They did not seem put off by the room. Despite their surroundings, or maybe because of them, my half-dozen participants worked very hard their first two days together, becoming a cohesive group and opening up to each other.

At the end of the second day, one of the group members invited us all to her apartment for dinner. Her home was a welcome change of scene from the spartan surroundings of the Glide basement. We had a nice long meal and after dinner went into her living room. She turned on a small radio, the music a pleasant backdrop to the animated conversation. Suddenly, the music stopped and a tense voice broke in:

"Broadcasting from the Ambassador Hotel . . ."

There followed a whoosh of static, then over the radio someone cried out.

"My god! My god. No! No!"

We sat in dumbfounded silence, staring at the radio. The voice came back to say that Senator Robert Kennedy had just been shot. He was bleeding from the head on the cement floor of the Ambassador Hotel kitchen. Mrs. Kennedy was with him. "Oh no, that poor family!" someone in our group said.

I felt stunned. Martin Luther King shot just two months ago, John Kennedy in Dallas. This was crazy. The announcer was back yelling almost hysterically into the microphone. Senator Kennedy had won the California presidential primary. He had just completed his victory speech and was leaving the Embassy Room through a kitchen corridor. He had stopped to shake hands with several of the kitchen staff when a man pointed a gun and began shooting. Kennedy was down, others were wounded, the shooter was grabbed. It all seemed to have happened in an instant. The announcer's words described a scene that was devastating and surreal.

That broadcast is frozen in my mind. We stayed with the radio for a while, hearing over and over again what had happened. Hardly anyone in our group spoke. People just sat transfixed, riveted on the radio. About

1 A.M., exhausted, we parted. I returned to my hotel shaken, unable to sleep, the words of the broadcast repeating in my brain.

The next morning at Glide Memorial Church, the seven chairs were pulled tightly into the smallest circle possible. It was as though we had drawn close to take comfort from one another's presence, protection from the mad, unpredictable world outside. We talked about the uncertainties of life and the profound effect that sudden death has on everyone's sense of equilibrium.

The morning and afternoon sessions were intense. When we left at the end of the day, Robert Kennedy's fate was still not known. When we gathered again on June 6, we knew that he had died in the night. The mood of the group was somber, and the talk was of vulnerability, which is what we were all feeling. I have never had a group experience like that one. I will never forget the Glide basement where seven who had been strangers were bonded by a distant tragedy and the impact of the unexpected.

CR∽ 13

In 1965, Watts exploded with the pent-up rage of black people frustrated by police brutality, dead-end lives, and the indifference of white society to their plight. Martin Luther King, Jr., said that riots are the voice of the unheard. The long scream in the night that rose up from Watts echoed across the nation.

"Burn, baby, burn!" the rioters chanted as they smashed windows, looted stores, and set fire to the neighborhoods. After five days of bloody warfare, thirty dead, hundreds injured, thousands arrested, the rioting was over and the governmental "fix" began. Federal money began to pour into the area. Some of the programs were helpful. Others were beside the point.

The main problem with Lyndon Johnson's War on Poverty was that it was fought on the wrong battlefield. Few people seemed to realize that what had to be "fixed" was not just the black ghetto but racist white America whose fear of change ensured that the ghetto would continue to restrict the movement of blacks into the mainstream. The programs that worked at all were those that created new opportunities for poor people to get the training they needed to become employable. I became involved in one of those programs.

I was hired by the California State Department of Rehabilitation to train indigenous aides to conduct groups with the hardcore unemployed in Watts. "Indigenous" meant that these aides were from the same neighborhoods as the people they would work with, the hope being that they could establish rapport with tough, resistant clients more easily than middle-class white professionals could. My mission was to teach aides the basics of how to run a group in which the clients could see themselves in action and identify the social and interpersonal difficulties they might encounter when they tried to get or hold onto jobs.

The training started with an intensive three-day retreat in a San Diego hotel. During the first two and a half days, the group members dealt with one another. They were comfortable doing that. On the last afternoon, I asked them to deal with me. I wanted them to witness a group leader being confronted because they would probably have to deal with such confrontation themselves in their own groups. They were not comfortable at all with that.

"Okay, if you won't tell me how you feel about me, I'll tell you what I feel about you," and I went around the group saying something to each person. That opened the door and one by one they ventured comments about me, all pretty mild stuff, polite, arm's length. I gave a little lecturette about being prepared to be challenged because most groups eventually do confront their leadership. They just looked at me. I reminded myself that I was not only the group leader here but also the only white person in the room, and I was not exactly giving them permission to deal with that particular salient fact. Did I even want to do that? I wasn't sure. I took the coward's way out and suggested we break for dinner.

When we assembled again in the meeting room I looked around and immediately saw that people had been drinking, some mildly boozed, others quite drunk. I realized that I'd made a terrible mistake not staying with the group for dinner. I had isolated myself and now I was more of an outsider than before. The fallout came quickly. One of the female aides spoke first.

"You know, you asked us before what we felt about you. Well I want to tell you now what I feel. Lady, you don't know jack shit about who we are or what we need."

"That's right," another chimed in, "you don't know jack shit."

A few group members shifted nervously in their chairs. I began to feel anxious. I sat very still. I was thinking about how to respond when I noticed a rather unnerving sound coming from one corner of the room. A group member named George was sitting on the edge of his chair and growling at me. The guttural sound seemed to come from deep inside him. He growled a few more times, then he stood up and started toward me. He was drunk and unsteady. George stopped about a foot in front of me. His eyes were red and watery. He leaned into my face and spoke almost inaudibly.

"Honky bitch!"

George's body was tense, his hands were tight fists against his sides.

"You are a honky bitch!" he said again, louder. "Honky bitch!"

I didn't move. My only thought was that they were right. I didn't know jack shit about this. I had no idea what might happen. Was I in danger? Would anyone in the room be my ally? I didn't know if I should stop him, call for help, or just sit there. My gut said just sit.

George stood in front of me, swaying slightly.

"Well," he said mostly to himself, "maybe I'm the man who can set this honky bitch straight."

That seemed to amuse him, and he began to laugh. He put his hands up to his head and laughed and laughed. Then abruptly, he stopped laughing. There was not a sound in the room, but I sensed that something different was happening. Slowly, I focused my eyes beyond George. I saw that three of the male group members had moved silently forward until they were inches behind George. They stood like statues, perfectly still, their arms outstretched, ready to grab him. But while he didn't move, they didn't move. We stayed in this strange tableau for several long minutes, like dancers frozen, waiting for some cue to resume motion. My heart was beating wildly, my hands were clammy, but I was determined not to move. I stared at George, and he stared back. Then, suddenly, his body began to shake as though it could no longer contain his anger. He let out a yell, and both his fists came up. The three men behind him lunged. They grabbed his arms, pulling him away from me, and wrestling him to the floor. I took a deep breath. When I tried to move, my body felt like it had turned to stone. The three aides walked George out of the room, and the others began to stir. Someone asked if I was okay and I found my voice enough to say I was.

"Cool," one of the group members said quietly. "You were cool."

Others nodded in agreement. I suggested we take a break then come back to talk about what had happened. As I stood up, several people approached and without a word put their arms around me. My body relaxed and those around me felt it. The barrier was down. By experiencing my vulnerability, the distance between us was reduced. They later told me that it was important to them that I'd not run away. White people usually run away from black anger. They thought I wasn't afraid, but of course I was. Despite my fear, I knew if I had run that would have been the end of me with them.

I survived the "honky bitch" crisis and had my head straightened out about how much I didn't know about what I was doing. That was my first awakening to the simmering hatred that underlay the race wars in America. It was not to be my last.

The violence in this country in 1968 seemed epidemic: the Robert Kennedy shooting, Martin Luther King, Jr., killed, and bloody riots in response to Dr. King's murder. Racial tensions were at an all-time high. I got a call from Dan Mermin, director of Bell & Howell's Human Development Institute in Atlanta. He wanted me to develop an ENCOUNTERTAPE program that would address the enmity between the races. The tapes could be used in grassroots settings without professional leaders. That meant that large numbers of people could go through a black/white encounter experience simultaneously.

I jumped at the chance to develop this program and was soon spending one week each month in Atlanta, writing, testing, revising group processes that we hoped would bring blacks and whites together to talk through their animosity. My coworker in this development phase was a young black man named Freeman T. Pollard. Freeman was twenty-six years old, big and broad shouldered, sweet, warm, funny, a charmer with a dazzling smile. At the drop of a hat, Freeman could be down-home country or he could be the ultimate sophisticate. He'd studied at Harvard and NYU, been a Peace Corps volunteer in Africa and a special assistant to the president of a southern college. Though I was fourteen years his senior, we easily established a peer relationship.

Freeman and I often worked in places away from the distractions of the busy HDI offices. On one of my trips, I was staying in a first-floor motel room with a large picture window that looked out on a walkway used by other guests. Freeman arrived, and we spread our papers out on the twin beds. We began working, but I noticed that Freeman seemed quite nervous. His head would swivel around to the window whenever anyone walked by. Finally I asked.

"Freeman, what on earth is wrong with you? What are you so antsy about?"

He glowered at me, shook his head, and finally said, "You don't get it, do you?"

"Get what?"

His tone had an edge to it. "You see, you are a white woman, I am a black man, and this is the South. We are alone in this motel room. Everyone who walks by sees that. Southern men do not take kindly to black men in motel rooms with white women. Sometimes they express themselves in very dramatic ways about this—like hauling my ass out of here and beating the shit out of me."

"But Freeman, we're just working in here. Anyone can see that."

Freeman shook his head.

"All these Southern crackers need to know is that a nigger is in here with a white lady."

Freeman walked over to the window and drew the drapes, then he turned and smiled, as though to reassure me that it was okay between us. We went back to work, but I was self-conscious after that. Maybe I was not the right person to be writing a race relations program. Maybe I still didn't know jack-shit enough.

The other person working with us was Dan Mermin, a white man and Freeman's best friend. It was Freeman's idea that the three of us should attend a race relations weekend workshop in San Francisco conducted by Price Cobbs, the black psychiatrist who wrote the book *Black Rage*. The brochure copy said the workshop would use the "bloodless riot" approach. I wondered what in the world that meant.

Price Cobbs had met Freeman and he knew who I was from my work at Esalen. There were about twenty people in the room, some black, some white. Price's four young black assistants sat unsmiling against one wall. To begin, Price talked about his conviction that the rationalizations and blindness that mask white racism had to be forcefully confronted before real dialogue between the races could take place. In the morning and the early afternoon, he talked about this issue, the "bloodless riot." In the late afternoon, he demonstrated his point—on me.

Price sat down right in front of me and began asking questions about my thinking on race relations. I was wary about his talking only to me, but I answered his questions. I'm improvising from memory here, but I believe I've got the tone right, if not Price's exact words. He began with several benign questions.

"What do you think whites want in their relations with blacks? Do you think most whites believe they are racists?"

Over the next hour, Price's questions became increasingly harsh and accusative. I tried to respond to him until, at one point, he stuck his face in mine and snarled, "Liar!" Price Cobbs was a big man with a powerful physique. He was so close to me I could feel the heat of his body. I wasn't sure what was happening. I felt confused, off-center. After calling me a liar numerous times, he began to shout in my face. I'm not sure what his words were, I just felt assaulted. Then he called upon his assistants to join in. They moved in on me in full force, shouting obscenities, their faces distorted with rage. Inches from me, they kept up a steady barrage. I didn't remember ever feeling so completely under attack.

I summoned all my courage and told them to leave me alone, but the words came out in a whisper and just seemed to make them angrier. They verbally pounded away at me, taunting, spitting out insults. I turned away, frightened, not sure what to do, but they moved with me, not letting up, allowing no retreat, no escape. "My god," I thought, "this is what Price Cobbs means by a goddam 'bloodless riot'?" I was trembling. All I could think of was getting away from these people, but there was no place to go. I was sitting on the floor, I backed up to the wall, and rolled myself into a ball, my hands covering my ears. I only wanted to cry but was determined not to. They kept on, pounding, pounding at me. Then, suddenly, Freeman was on his feet rushing at Price and the other four.

"Leave her alone! Damn it, leave her alone!"

Everything stopped dead.

Price approached Freeman, who now stood by himself in the middle of the room.

"Well, well, what have we here?" Price said, coyly. "A black man who rescues white women?"

Freeman mumbled something about it being unnecessary to be so brutal. Then he looked like he was sorry he'd said anything at all. Price put his face up very close to Freeman's. Slowly and deliberately he hissed, "What we seem to have here is a black man with natural hair but a processed mind."

Freeman said nothing. He stood frozen to the spot, his eyes following Price who was circling him. There was silence in the room. Then Price stopped in front of Freeman and said slowly into his face, "You have some work to do, brother. You need to find out what your priorities are. You need to do something about that processed mind. Now sit down and try to get with the program."

Freeman sat. Price came over to where I was still rolled up against the wall. He got on his knees and spoke into my ear, loudly enough so the whole room could hear,

"You see, this is what it's like to be black in America. White folks get up in your face and they call you names and swear at you and insult you. You say stop but they go right on. They don't care how you feel or what it's doing to you. They want you to be scared to death so you can't defy them. They want you to be all rolled up like this, harmless and neutralized. This is my message. If you want to fight in our war, you damn well better know how it feels to be black in this country, every day, every night, everywhere you go, your whole life long. This battle is never over. You can't quit and you can't escape. That's what you have to get, the relentlessness of it. If you don't get that you don't get anything!"

Price slowly backed away. I said nothing and I didn't move. Price ended the session and said he'd see us the next morning. People got up slowly, quietly, and filed out.

Freeman and Dan came to me and gently lifted me to my feet. I felt unsteady. None of us spoke as we walked to the car, but once I was in the backseat, the dam burst for me and I cried, wracking sobs that released the feelings I'd been holding in for an hour. Freeman reached back and held my hand. Then, suddenly, something happened, the reason for which I have never really understood. Maybe it was the heightened emotionality of the afternoon, triggering the need in all of us for release. Freeman turned to Dan, who was driving, and he choked out Dan's name, as though to get his attention. Dan looked perplexed.

"What, Freeman, what?"

"You know I'm gay, don't you Dan? You do know that, don't you?"

Dan looked at Freeman disbelievingly. The car swerved. Dan quickly returned his eyes to the road.

"I've wanted to tell you for so long," Freeman went on. "I don't know why I'm telling you now, but I don't want to hold it back any more."

Dan looked straight ahead but said, "Okay, Freeman. I didn't know, but I'm glad you told me."

I couldn't believe this was happening. I'd been afraid to tell Freeman I was gay because I was worried about what he would think of me. I put my hand on his shoulder and I could hardly get the words out. "Freeman, I'm gay too."

Now it was Freeman's turn to look disbelieving. He turned to me. "You are?"

I nodded and Freeman reached back and grabbed my hand again, squeezing it hard. Freeman, so different from me in so many ways—in different decades of our lives, different gender, different race, but suddenly we had something so much in common that it seemed to obliterate all the other differences.

In the hotel elevator, Dan put his arms around his longtime friend and with that he didn't have to say anything. Freeman smiled and looked relieved. These two would remain the closest of friends, even more strongly bonded by this extraordinary day than they had been before.

We ordered dinner in Dan and Freeman's room, not wanting to be apart. We talked about what had happened, and we all agreed that Price Cobbs's approach to racial encounter was too strong an approach for our audiotape-directed groups. It had been too strong for me. I was still shaky inside, and I kept thinking what did I do to deserve such treatment. And no doubt that is exactly what Price Cobbs wanted me to think because that is the question that lies at the heart of the pain for black people in white racist America.

As I was leaving to return to my room, Freeman said, "Are you going back tomorrow?"

"I don't know. Are you?"

Freeman looked straight at me. "I have no choice," he said. "I have to go back."

I, too, went back the next day, but I didn't say a single word. Price avoided me. I listened and watched, and I was glad when it was over. That night, Freeman, Dan, and I flew to Los Angeles. On Monday morning, Price Cobbs phoned me. "Are you all right?" he asked. "You were pretty quiet yesterday."

For a moment, I thought about telling him that I was not all right, using his concern to punish him for his brutal treatment of me, but I didn't.

"I'm fine," I said.

"Good. I'm glad. Well, let me know if I can be helpful to you in any way. Be seeing you."

As it turned out, we did see each other quite soon. The following month, Price turned up on a racism panel with me at the University of Georgia. Here was the cool intellectual Price Cobbs, calmly discussing race relations issues. As I watched him, I could see his snarling face an inch from mine, screaming at me, "Liar! Liar! Liar!" I would never forget the lesson of his bloodless riot. I would never forget him.

Freeman, Dan, and I finished the *Black/White ENCOUNTERTAPES*, and they were used for years in a variety of situations where race relations were an issue, particularly in the military. Freeman and I remained friends, staying in touch during the long periods when he lived and worked in Africa, seeing each other when he returned to this country. In 1987 we went together to the National March for Lesbian and Gay Rights in Washington. Freeman died of AIDS in 1991. Dan Mermin gave the eulogy at his memorial service.

It was my last night in Atlanta. I was having dinner with John, one of the HDI staff members. After dinner John asked if there was any place I'd like to go. It occurred to me that I would like to see where Martin Luther King, Jr., was buried, so I asked John if he knew where the grave was.

"No idea," he said, "but it shouldn't be hard to find out."

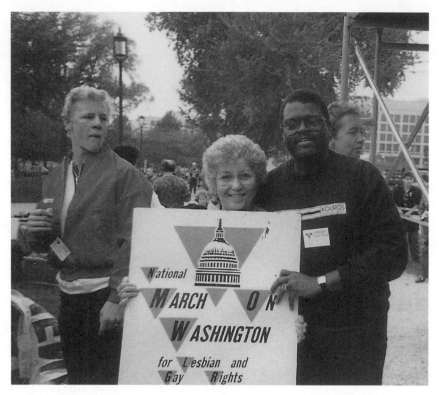

Freeman Pollard, my colleague and friend from the Human Development Institute in Atlanta and my coauthor of the *Black/White ENCOUNTERTAPES*. We are in Washington, D.C., at the 1987 March for Lesbian and Gay Rights.

We drove to one of Atlanta's black neighborhoods. John went into a convenience store and asked directions to Dr. King's burial place. No one in the store knew where it was. We drove on until we saw two people walking down the street. I rolled down my window and asked if they knew where Dr. King was buried. Both shrugged, they didn't know. John pulled into a gas station. Nope, no one there had any idea where the grave was.

I couldn't believe it. How could people not know this.

Then I had an idea. I went to a telephone and called a taxi. When it arrived, I asked the question. Sure, the driver knew where the burial site was—South View Cemetery in south Atlanta. We hired the cab and followed it to a rather desolate area of town. The gates to the South View Cemetery were closed, and I assumed at such a late hour they would be locked, but

I got out of the car anyway and pushed on the gates. To my astonishment they swung open.

Inside the dark cemetery, we drove slowly along a narrow winding road. About two hundred yards down the road, we saw a white canopy over a crypt with a small flame burning in front of it. That had to be it. We stopped and got out. The night was very still. Standing in front of the crypt, in the flickering light of the flame, we read the words engraved there.

"Free at last, free at last, thank God Almighty, I'm free at last."

I felt in awe to be in such close proximity to this extraordinary man. I contemplated the words, beginning to blur through tears as I thought about the tragedy of Dr. King's death, the loss to so many people whose lives he might yet have touched. When I looked up, I couldn't believe what I saw. Just beyond the crypt, across the narrow street and quite visible from where we stood, were a neon-lit gas station and a laundromat. Several cars went by. How unseemly a last resting place for a man of such distinction, a Nobel Prize winner, an inspired leader, a giant among human beings. It seemed too undignified, too accessible. But he wouldn't be there for long.

Later, I learned that Dr. King had been interred initially at South View because his grandparents were buried there. In 1970 he was moved to the newly constructed Martin Luther King, Jr., Center for Nonviolent Social Change in Atlanta. His crypt stands on a raised platform in the middle of a sizable reflecting pool, a much more fitting burial site for Martin Luther King, Jr., much more suitable for this great man than an unlocked cemetery across the street from a gas station and a laundromat. It is said that a million people a year visit the center to pay their respects to Dr. King, standing before the reflecting pool, viewing his crypt from that distance. But at one o'clock in the morning in June 1969, he was resting in that unlocked cemetery, and we stood alone with him in the quiet summer night.

14

In 1971, Bell & Howell, having suffered financial losses in some of their product lines, closed my office as an economy measure. I was on my own, eased out by a generous severance package. I started to edit a book on encounter groups with Larry Solomon and I stepped up my workshop schedule. I was living in the first house I'd ever owned, a tiny two-bedroom aerie high in the Hollywood Hills above the Sunset Strip. Because the house was on stilts, I enjoyed a thrilling view from downtown to the ocean. It was not so thrilling on February 9, however, when everything at 8560 Hollywood Boulevard began to shimmy and shake.

The house rocked and rolled, the glassware fell out of the cabinets, the pictures slid off the walls, the furniture skidded across the floor, and light fixtures came crashing down from the ceiling. Through the rattling windows I could see transformers all over the city exploding in brilliant blue arcs. I was frozen with fright and sure the house would topple over and end up in the street below. I was certainly going to die.

The 6.6 earthquake and the aftershocks continued into the next day, but the house didn't fall down. There is something about being betrayed by the ground underneath you that feels like the ultimate treachery. It took weeks to regain my equilibrium. I was reassured by the former owner and builder of the house, who sent me detailed drawings of how the house was supported—sixteen steel and concrete columns set ten feet into bedrock. The house was designed to swing and sway in an earthquake but not fall down. For the next twelve years that little hill house was my home. After the next major quake in 1994, when I no longer lived there, I took the drawings to the occupant of 8560 Hollywood Boulevard, who was as grateful as I had been to receive them.

"Why bother?" Roberto demanded. Roberto was my buddy, my mainstay, as I explored the possibilities for meeting other lesbians. Roberto accompanied me to lesbian bars that made me so nervous that I looked at no one, talked to no one, and never left Roberto's side.

"What is it with you? Do you want to be a lesbian or don't you?" he asked.

"Of course I want to be—I am a lesbian."

"Then why don't you act like one. Women here are cruising you, but you just look away!"

I didn't understand it any more than he did. I just couldn't get comfortable in this environment. I said, "I never went to bars to meet men when I was being heterosexual. It doesn't feel anymore right to go to a bar to meet a woman."

"Bullshit! I don't think that's the problem at all. You had a relationship behind closed doors with someone who didn't even think of herself as lesbian. You didn't have to be gay in life. Now you do, that's what you're so scared about, really being a lesbian."

He was right, of course. The problem was that the many years of defining my attraction to women as dangerous ground had taken their toll. I had trained myself to turn off to women I was attracted to. In these bars I felt drawn to practically everybody, but I could not overcome the anxiety I felt about sexual feelings toward women. I just shut down to be safe, and so far I'd not found a way to retrieve myself from this limbo. Bars seemed not to be the answer.

Why didn't gay people have a variety of places to meet and socialize just as straight people did? It seemed unfair that gays had only bars to go to. I felt irritated about being told, in essence, that my access to other gays could only happen where straight society decided it was all right. Maybe it was time to change all this. I had, after all, brought hundreds of straights together in my Quest for Love workshops. Why not do the same for gays? Would they come? I'd heard that homosexuals had put on a parade the previous summer, walking right down the middle of Hollywood Boulevard carrying signs saying they were gay and proud. Wouldn't that mean there were some who would come to a gay growth center? I started talking to people about it.

A psychologist friend referred me to a community psychiatrist at UCLA, Martin Field, who was meeting with a group of gay activists who wanted to open a gay social services center. I discovered that, yes, Dr. Field was consulting with such a group, and yes, he would be glad to introduce me to them. He would bring them over to my house.

167

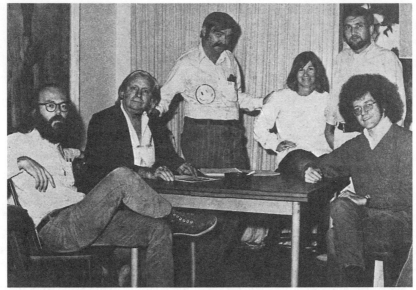

FIRST PORTRAIT. Officers and directors of Los Angeles' Gay Community Services Center meet to discuss the acquisition and opening of the Center's new home, a 10-room Victorian mansion. They are, from left: Executive Director Don Kilhefner, Vice President Morris Kight, gay activist Jim Kepner, social worker June Herrle. President Martin Field. a UCLA psvchiatrist. and management analvst John Platania.

1971, after I moved to Los Angeles to explore being gay an odd little group came to me to talk about opening a community center for gays. They met in my living room over the summer. In October the Gay Community Services Center opened, the first of its kind anywhere.

I had never met an activist before. Now I wondered what I was getting into. Images of bomb-throwing Bolsheviks came to mind. "That's stupid," I told myself, "middle-class paranoia working overtime! UCLA psychiatrists didn't consult with bomb-throwing Bolsheviks." On July 7, 1971, I opened the door of my home to an oddly assorted little band of people who would enter my life and change its direction forever.

They trooped in single file, looking about as apprehensive of me as I was of them. First came Don Kilhefner in workshirt, construction boots, scraggly beard, long hair, glasses. John Platania was a sight to behold; his oversized red Afro framed his face like a halo. He glided in, shimmering white shirt and harem trousers flowing gently around him. June Herrle was a rather ordinary-looking young woman, jeans and T-shirt. Jim Kepner, older, unsmiling, with eyes that looked as though they had already seen too much.

Morris Kight, middle-aged, kindly round face, longish blond hair going gray, an air of authority about him. Martin Field brought up the rear.

As though it was the expected thing, Morris spoke first. "Now, my dear Miss Berzon . . . ," he began and proceeded to deliver a flowery oration that included the history of gay liberation, how it related to the struggles of other oppressed groups in the world, why the planet was in dire peril, and what we all needed to do about it. His presentation was eloquent, and I was enchanted. As he wound down, he finally began to talk about the plans his group had for a gay community center.

At this point others began to chime in. June, who was a social worker, saw the center as a place where gays could get counseling and other social services. The men were particularly interested in assisting gay males who had been arrested for "sexual misconduct," given that such arrests in those days often involved police entrapment. Their plan was to intervene on behalf of the accused in court and to make their own "rehabilitation programs" available to ease the conditions of probation. Educating heterosexuals in the helping professions was of interest to all of them. And there were other legal, medical, personal-growth, and cultural programs they had ideas about. In their enthusiasm, they talked over and around one another.

I was amazed at the scope of their vision and the grandiosity of their plans. Kilhefner and Kight were quite sure they could raise money among wealthy homosexuals and get funding for their project from a variety of government agencies and private foundations. As I listened I thought how incredibly naive they seemed. What government official would stick out a civil-service neck to fund a homosexual organization? What wealthy gay person would risk exposure by becoming involved with this maverick group? Didn't they understand how powerless they were, how innocent, how vulnerable? I feared for their safety and their sanity in undertaking this project. Nevertheless, I offered to help them by designing a growth-group program and by training peer counselors to run the groups. They were delighted.

In the months ahead, I met often with these people, and it was I who got quite an education. I came to see that they were neither powerless, naive, nor innocent. In fact, they were incredibly resourceful, persistent, and clever, as practical in their strategies as they were passionate in their advocacy. Tradition, convention, the law itself were up for grabs as these people plowed past obstacles to achieve the impossible—establishment of the first community center and social service agency designed to meet the needs of homosexual men and women. I still thought they were crazy, but I was hooked. Working with them was one of the most exciting things I'd ever done.

I watched in amazement as Kilhefner, Kight, and company pressed on in the face of unabashed hostility from bureaucrats, law enforcement, and social service agencies. They used guerilla tactics to get around regulations they couldn't possibly comply with. They scrounged equipment and furniture they couldn't possibly buy. By some miracle, or so it seemed to me, they pirated a telephone system, rented a building, got permits, and set up their operation. Their schemes were brilliant and outrageous and they worked. I was in awe of their chutzpah and their unflagging commitment. They simply did not take no for an answer, from anyone, about anything.

On the afternoon of October 16, 1971, I stood on the sidewalk and looked at the ten-room, falling-down wreck of a Victorian mansion on Wilshire Boulevard with the sign right out front for all the world to see: GAY COMMUNITY SERVICES CENTER. Never before had there been such a sign or such a place. I felt proud to have had something to do with this extraordinary venture.

On October 16, the Center's first day of life, people streamed through the building, most looking as astonished as I felt. There were members of the Los Angeles City Council, the few movers and shakers of the nascent gay rights movement, the Center's small board of directors, volunteers, friends of the founders, and the press. Over the next two years, many thousands of people would use the Center's counseling and consciousness-raising groups, housing, employment, legal aid, probation and parole services, and medical and STD clinics. As planned, volunteer lawyers, physicians, and nurses participated in the programs, but I had insisted that the counseling program be run on a peer-counselor basis. For the next four years I trained dozens of nonprofessionals to run various kinds of growth groups at the Center.

Deciding to get involved with the formation of the Gay and Lesbian Community Services Center (as it was subsequently called) was one of the best things I ever did for myself. In that first year I spent hours in conversation with Don Kilhefner and Morris Kight, both dedicated activists with long experience on the front lines of civil rights movements. They understood how anger and advocacy interacted, fed off one another, and created opportunities for unprecedented change. Through Kilhefner and Kight I was able to achieve a clarity about what it means to be gay that I'd never had. I came to see that we were a community just forming, a powerful force just barely beginning to stir itself. For the first time in my life I was having positive feelings about an aspect of myself that I had spent decades in turn denying and hating myself for.

In the early 1970s I began doing speaking engagements for the Center, talking about what homosexuality means, who gay people are, and the Center's mission. I grew close to many of the young people in my training classes, and I always took three or four of them with me whenever I spoke publicly. They talked about their gay lives while I talked about homosexuality in the abstract. It took about six months for them finally to confront me.

"Do you realize that when anyone in the audience asks if you are gay, you have a five, a ten, and a fifteen minute answer in none of which you say you are gay?"

"I don't think so. I always say I'm gay."

In chorus they shouted at me, "Never! You never say you're gay!"

I was flabbergasted. I protested, but my young friends would not let me get away with that denial. The next few speaking engagements, when the question was inevitably asked, "Are you gay?" they would lean forward in unison and scrutinize me. I couldn't get the words out fast enough. "Yes, I *am* gay." It became clear that the coming out process is never over. There are always new disclosure challenges, and young activists then, as now, did not hesitate to hold one's feet to the fire. So, I trained them and they trained me. We were mutually transforming ourselves.

September 1971. One of the things I was looking forward to at the annual meetings of the American Psychological Association in Washington, D.C., was getting together with a San Francisco psychologist I had become acquainted with by telephone but whom I had never met. His name was Don Clark, and he initially contacted me because he was writing a report on the Human Potential Movement for the Carnegie Foundation. It was soon revealed in our conversations that we were both just coming out as gay. Don was still married and living with his wife and children, but he had already begun to speak publicly as a gay man and was writing a book, *Loving Someone Gay.*

When we met, it turned out that Don felt as I did, that we should try to do something to raise consciousness about being gay within the profession of psychology. We could start right there at APA. Why not simply call a meeting of the gay and lesbian psychologists attending the convention? We looked at each other and laughed. In 1971, who was going to admit to being a gay psychologist by coming to such a meeting? No one, that's who.

"Let's do it anyway," Don said. "What is there to lose?"

I agreed. We both felt secure enough with our own professional status, and we were both convinced that the time had come for pushing a little further out of the closet. We decided to publicize our improbable event by putting up signs around the half-dozen APA convention hotels. We went from floor to floor in our hotel stealing laundry bags from the housekeeping carts. Using magic markers to make our signs, we announced:

"Meeting of Gay and Lesbian Members of APA in Room 615, Washington Hilton, Friday at 6:00 P.M."

Like thieves in the night, we went stealthily from hotel to hotel, looking over our shoulders each time we hurriedly attached a laundry bag to a corridor wall. When it was over, we felt exhilarated.

On Friday afternoon at 5:30 Don and I met in my room. We sat stiffly on one of the twin beds, nervously eyeing the door.

"What do you think will happen?" Don asked.

"Nothing, I imagine," I said. "We'll just sit here like fools and nobody will come and then we'll go out to dinner and comfort each other for being so silly as to think we could do this."

"Right," he said. "You're probably right."

At exactly six o'clock there was a knock on the door. Don and I looked at each other. For a moment I thought neither of us was going to answer it. Then Don walked slowly to the door and opened it. Two people stood outside, a man and a woman.

"Come in," Don said.

They came in, looking around cautiously. We introduced ourselves. Another knock at the door, then another, and another. Within fifteen minutes there were twenty-five people in the room. Several were psychologists I knew, and we greeted each other with sly smiles.

After a while, I stood up on a chair and got everyone's attention. The first meeting ever of gay and lesbian psychologists was underway. I will never forget the sight of that crowd, lying across beds, sitting on the floor, leaning against the wall, every inch of space taken, men and women courageous enough, or maybe just ready enough, to risk exposure that could be professionally damaging to assert their need to be known for who they really were.

We discussed ways of exchanging experiences on what it was like to be a gay professional in the university, social service agency, or clinical practice. We brainstormed gay-themed research projects that might get funded by private foundations. It was wonderfully exciting to be speaking this way, as though doing so was a bold step into the open. After several hours, we wound down and started talking about getting together again. Don and I invited people to write to either of us if they wanted to be part of the "network," and we wrote our own addresses on one of the laundry bags and attached it to the wall. There was high energy in the room. People exchanged addresses with one another. They thanked us for making the impromptu meeting happen. Many of us went to dinner together, continuing to talk, wanting to hang onto the feeling of freedom and openness that had started in that hotel room.

The convention ended and we returned to our workplaces. The exhilaration of the evening soon faded into memory. We had purposely not taken people's names and addresses because we didn't want them to feel threatened. What a stupid mistake! We realized later that we had allowed our own homophobia to deprive us of an opportunity for staying in touch with everyone. How dumb we were, how co-opted by rules designed to keep us isolated from one another! A few people wrote to us, but not enough to think of organizing something for next year's convention. As it happened, the following year both Don and I attended the Association for Humanistic Psychology meetings in Squaw Valley rather than the APA convention.

At the 1972 APA meetings—I like to think it was because of the seeds we had sown—a group of gay and lesbian psychologists protested an APA panel on homosexuality consisting entirely of heterosexuals. The chairperson of the panel had announced that there were no gay psychologists on the panel because he had no knowledge of any admittedly gay psychologists within APA and he was not willing to request that any psychologist jeopardize his or her career by appearing as a homosexual. That did it. A core group of five young gay psychologists met that evening and out of their rage at what had happened in the afternoon symposium formulated the idea for the Association of Gay Psychologists.

In 1973, the American Psychological Association sponsored their first formal symposium on homosexuality in which the panel was made up *entirely* of openly gay and lesbian psychologists. Was anyone interested in what they had to say? Four hundred people attended the session. The conspiracy of silence around gays and lesbians in the APA was broken forever.

January 1972. Don Clark and I have put together a panel for the California State Psychological Association annual meeting, the first openly gay panel ever to present at a psychological convention. As Don and I approached the

Ambassador Hotel on that sunny Saturday afternoon, we both felt nervous. Once again, we wondered if anyone would respond to us. We had talked at lunch about dire possibilities—we could be ridiculed, heckled, ostracized, or just ignored. It felt as though we were stepping off a precipice, but we squared our shoulders and marched heads up into the corridor leading to our meeting room. There was a commotion around the doorway to our room. Trouble already? My stomach was in knots.

We pushed our way through the crowd at the door. Inside, it was wall-to-wall people, many more than the room was meant to hold, and they were three deep in the doorway. We made our way to the front. People were sitting on the floor all around the podium. A row of tape recorders faced us on the table. Our fellow panelists were already seated, looking wide-eyed as even more people pushed their way into the crowded room.

At exactly two o'clock, Don stood and began to speak. One by one, we talked about the experience of being gay and of working professionally with gay men and women. After each panel member spoke, there was prolonged applause, as though the audience was applauding not just the presentation but the fact of our being there at all. When it was over, many people crowded around us, saying things that made me feel gratified that we had done this.

"I'm gay and I never imagined I would attend a symposium like this."

"I'm gay and I've never told that to a stranger before."

"I'm gay and I feel okay about it for the first time ever today."

The year 1973 was a banner year for confrontation between gay activists and the mental health establishment. A particularly aggressive group of East Coast gays worked long and hard lobbying the leadership of the American Psychiatric Association to drop homosexuality from its list of mental illnesses. Their names should be prominent in any roll call of heroes of the gay rights movement: Frank Kameny, Barbara Gittings, Ron Gold, Bruce Voeller, Howard Brown, and Charles Silverstein. The deed was finally done on December 15, 1973, thus effecting the quickest cure in history. In what might be considered something of a run on liberating proclamations, the APA resolution freeing homosexuals from the stigma of mental illness occurred the same year the Pope declared that the Jews were no longer to be blamed for the death of Christ. It would take the American Psychological Association another year to follow the lead of the American Psychiatric Association, declaring in January 1975 that homosexuality was not a mental disorder and deploring discrimination against gays in the public and private sectors.

Professionally, I continued to edge out into public view. Inspired by the success of the California State Psychological Association symposium, I negotiated with UCLA to present their first official program for the public on the topic of homosexuality. June 21, 1972, several hundred people gathered for an all-day symposium titled "The Homosexual in America." The panel included a psychiatrist (enlightened), an attorney (gay legal issues), Dr. Evelyn Hooker, Morris Kight, Don Kilhefner, and three young gay activists—including Rand Schrader, a law student (later an openly gay judge). A measure of the success of this symposium was the document signed by most of the participants at the end of the day petitioning UCLA to sponsor additional programs on the topic of homosexuality.

It was only a glimmer so far, but gay visibility was beginning to happen, sometimes in unexpected and truly memorable ways. I will never forget the chill down my back as I watched the platform committee sessions of the Democratic Convention on television in the summer of 1972. One o'clock in the morning, a tall, thin young man takes the podium, looks directly into the camera, and says to America, "My name is Jim Foster and I am a gay man."

I sat bolt upright in bed. In 1972 that was a stunner. Jim Foster was speaking in favor of a gay rights plank in the party platform. It would take twenty more years before another gay man, Bob Hattoy, would step up to the podium to address the Democratic Convention and the nation as an openly gay man, not at one o'clock in the morning, but in prime time.

My personal evolution as a lesbian was not keeping up with my progress as a gay activist. While I was now meeting lesbian women, none of these contacts ripened into anything romantic. I tended to blame this on the "imperfect" people I was encountering, continuing to be out of touch with how defended I was against emotional involvement as a lesbian.

It was a sunny summer Sunday at the beach. Roberto and I were drinking beer at a local pub. "Don't look now," he said, "but that blonde at the bar is cruising you."

I looked. The "blonde at the bar" was either Candace Bergen or her twin. "Impossible," I said. "No one who looks like that would be cruising me!"

"Look again."

Yes, this gorgeous woman was definitely staring at me. She smiled. I smiled back. Soon she joined us at our table. She was not Candace Bergen, but she could have been her twin. Though she had feminine good looks, her nickname was Butch. In her twenties she had lived with her husband, a gay man, in a charade of a marriage. They were both quite proud of having fooled their middle-class families with an elaborate wedding, after which they went off on honeymoons with their respective lovers.

Butch was not interested in a romance with me, but for some reason she took it upon herself to take charge of my social life. She knew hundreds of lesbians and she introduced me to all of them. Most were young, in their twenties and thirties, a few were my own age. They were the vanguard of what would later be called "lipstick lesbians"—attractive, fashionable clothes, cars, and apartments, fast-track lives, good jobs, and always up for a good time.

At Butch's behest, I gave a series of parties at my Hollywood Hills home that, I'm told, people still talk about. I supplied the food and the booze, Butch did the inviting, and for a while my house on Saturday night was the hottest lesbian hangout in town. There were times when several hundred women were in attendance. They crowded into every room, down the stair-well, and out onto the two decks. Sometimes I worried that the house would slide down the hill with all those people in it, but it had survived the earth-quake, so I figured it would probably survive the lesbians.

So here they were: dozens of women in my house, mine to choose from—well, not quite. They were very interested in my parties. They were not par-ticularly interested in me. I tried to connect with these lesbians, but I seemed to have so little in common with them. The good news of gay liberation had not reached them. They seemed to have few interests beyond gossip, clothes, restaurants, trips, and their latest love affairs.

I tried desperately to fit in, but I felt like my nose was pressed up against the window of their lives as it had once been pressed against the window of Terry's Bar in Greenwich Village. These were not the sad, isolated lesbians of the '40s and '50s, but in a strangely similar way they also seemed out of it—too absorbed in their personal dramas to be in touch with what was happening in the world around them. Though I saw their lives as shallow and their interests as superficial, I kept trying to be accepted by them.

I stayed with this scene longer than I should have, probably because I had convinced myself that there was something wrong with me. Why couldn't I loosen up and be like them? I tried to do that by drinking, but that only brought out the underlying hostility I felt toward these people. My annoy-ance with them, which I didn't even acknowledge as such, ensured distance.

Any attempt I thought I was making with these women to accept and enjoy being a lesbian was an exercise in futility. It was the wrong crowd.

Gradually, I retrieved myself, withdrew from Butch and her minions, and with relief, turned back to the much more exciting and compatible company of my activist friends. Once again, I was reminded of the danger of trying to be something I was not. I had spent so much of my life doing that, trying to be like other people, to be "normal." I didn't even know what "normal" was anymore, but one thing was clear, every time I went outside myself for a definition of who I was, I ended up lost and off the compass.

"I'm going to die," Roberto said.

"Come on, what do you mean you're going to die?"

"I'm dying of cancer."

I felt the smile fading from my face. I was visiting Roberto in the hospital where he'd gone for tests after discovering a large bump on his head. Roberto was a kidder, and I wasn't ready yet to believe he was telling me the truth.

"What kind of cancer do you have?"

"Bone. They think that's how it started, but it's all through my body now. There's nothing they can do."

I couldn't believe what I was hearing. "Roberto, is this a joke?"

"No, it's true, I'm going to die."

I asked him to tell me everything the doctor had said, which wasn't much beyond the awful prognosis that Roberto repeated over and over. Then he cried, and I held him and cried with him. It felt as though a large dark hole had opened up and swallowed us both.

When he was hospitalized I went to see him every day, always fearing what I would see when I got there, wondering if I would be able to handle it. I took my cue from Roberto; when he was in good humor, we'd gossip and laugh. Sometimes he'd want to be quiet, and then we'd watch television together, not needing to say anything.

Every day Roberto grew weaker. His mood fluctuated from sadness to anger to great calm. On the days when he was feeling better, he took delight in phoning people he knew in Los Angeles and New York, telling them quite casually that he was dying of cancer and that there was something he had been wanting to say to them. Then he would tell them exactly what he thought was wrong with their lives and what he thought they should do about it. Some of these people never did believe his opening statement and were so offended they hung up on him. He didn't seem to care. He was enjoying enormously his freedom to say whatever he wanted without worrying about future consequences.

Roberto got special care at Cedars of Lebanon Hospital, where he'd been a respiratory therapist while pursuing his acting career. He was well-liked by his fellow workers there, and the nurses were attentive to his every need. Though he could not afford one, he was given a private room as a courtesy. Friends visited, then fell away as he got sicker, until there were only three of us left: Joe, an old friend from New York, Shirley, a young nurse he'd been close to while working at the hospital, and me.

In the fourth week of his hospitalization, I learned what my special assignment was to be. Roberto had been orphaned as an infant when his parents were killed in a car crash; he'd been raised by an uncle. Since he'd left Honduras at eighteen, he'd had little contact with his family. He saw no reason to have a funeral or burial, so he gave his body to a medical school. He did, however, want to be memorialized, and that was my job. I was to throw a wonderful party for him at my house. He told me exactly what kind of food he wanted served and what music he wanted played, and he provided the entire guest list. I told him I would do exactly as he wished.

In the fifth week, Roberto was too weak to leave his bed. He was being heavily sedated on morphine, and he would drift in and out of coherence. Once, as I sat by his bed, he opened his eyes and tried to sit up. He called me by a name I'd never heard.

"Chita, let's go out and play," he said. "It's such a pretty day. Take my hand, I'll show you where we can go." He lay there smiling. Then he began to speak softly in Spanish, and I knew he was back in Honduras in his childhood and I was one of his little cousins. I took his hand and held it until he fell asleep.

On Thursday of the fifth week, as I was leaving, I had to tell Roberto I wouldn't see him for a few days, until Sunday, because I had to do the California State Psychological Association presentation. I felt horrible saying it. How could I not be with him in these last days of his life? What could be that important? He just smiled at me.

"It's okay," he said, "see ya."

Silently, I asked Roberto to wait for me, not to die until I could be with him, but he wasn't able to wait. Late Friday afternoon, Shirley called.

"Roberto died," she said quietly. I was devastated. He was thirty-three years old. He'd hardly lived his life. How unfair, how crazy. Why did this have to happen to him . . . to me? He was my soul mate, my confidant, my hedge against loneliness. I needed him. I felt lost without him.

"Take my hand. I'll show you where we can go."

He always led me. He was doing it again with his party. Though I was heavy with sadness, on Sunday afternoon my gift to Roberto got underway. I served the food he had ordered and played the music he requested. Everyone on the list showed up, people from all parts of Roberto's life, come to mourn, laugh, cry, and share remembrances of him. Then I, too, received a gift on this day. Roberto's friend Phil had called to say he couldn't come to the party because his dog was about to have puppies. I told him it was okay, but several hours later Phil appeared. He said he had to come for just a few minutes. Phil was a teacher, a sweet, gentle person. When he left the party, he went out the door, then came back.

"Would you like one of the puppies?"

"Yes," I said immediately, though I'd never had a pet in my life. After Phil left I realized I hadn't asked what kind of dog it was— what if it was a St. Bernard, an English sheep dog? Fortunately, Raggy turned out to be a small Australian terrier. He was to be my constant companion for the next fifteen years, feisty, independent, charming, and fun, just like Roberto. And, like Roberto, he resisted all attempts to tame his natural exuberance to the demands of obedience, but I didn't care. I adored him, even when he embarrassed me by mounting the leg of every male friend who came through the front door. I'd yell at the little humper, "Stop!" But he never did. I was certain that Roberto lived in that dog.

15

"What are *you* doing here?" I demanded.

Sheldon laughed, "What are *you* doing here?"

In January 1973 I joined the Board of Directors of the Gay Community Services Center. At my first meeting I was shocked to see Sheldon Andelson, a man I had dated in my "heterosexual" life, neither of us having arrived at the truth quite yet in those days. We were delighted to have found one another in this new incarnation. Sheldon and I would spend many community meetings together over the next decade and a half.

I write about Sheldon here because he is a prime example of an openly gay man who became enormously powerful in the mainstream world. Sheldon's wealth came not only from his thriving law practice but from his extensive real estate holdings. He had quietly been buying up West Hollywood property long before that colorful neighborhood became the center of the city's gay and lesbian population.

In the 1980s Sheldon opened the Bank of Los Angeles and Trumps, one of the city's most successful restaurants for the next dozen years. Sheldon was also active in state and national politics and became an acknowledged behind-the-scenes power broker in the Democratic Party. Appointed by Governor Jerry Brown to the University of California Board of Regents, Sheldon's nomination sparked a grueling battle with the California legislature, going through six ballots before he was confirmed. He was justifiably proud when he won because he stood up to formidable opposition as an openly gay man and never backed down.

Through his political connections, Sheldon brought many members of the gay and lesbian community into positions of influence as judges, commissioners, and elected officials. He was a person who made things happen, not always to everyone's liking (Sheldon had his supporters and his detractors), but no one can deny that he was an important force in building clout for gays and lesbians in Los Angeles and throughout California. He raised the bar on what is possible to achieve as an openly gay person in our society. Sheldon would be an integral part of my life for many years to come.

It was a beautiful summer day in the lushly green, wooded splendor of Topanga Canyon, where life was simple and rustic and the air was washed clear by the breezes from the Pacific Ocean. In June 1973, I was conducting a gay Quest for Love weekend at the Topanga Human Development Center, hoping this time some women would show up. One did, along with eight gay men.

I watched the tall woman descend the stairs from the street above. So this was the lone lesbian. She was attractive, hair in a Jane Fonda shag, gray denim suit, nice eyes, not my type. I began the group with introductions. The woman in gray spoke and I looked away, aware of a feeling of embarrassment. What in the world? Was I embarrassed to look at her? Not this same old stuff again, surely. Would I ever relax enough to be able to look directly at an attractive woman? Was I going to spend the rest of my life learning how to be a lesbian?

Introductions completed, we moved into the plan for the day. I set up the first exercise, in which group members had to choose a partner. Half the men wanted to pair up with the woman in gray, and she ended up with a young man in his late twenties, about her age I guessed. She seemed quite at ease with men, obviously not a lesbian at odds with the opposite sex. By midmorning I had begun working more intensively with group members in various combinations. I paid attention to all the men, but I ignored the woman. I was appalled at my behavior, and I wondered whether anyone in the group was noticing.

That night I confronted myself. How outrageous of me to ignore a group member who had come in good faith to my workshop. Why was I so threatened by this person? I seemed to have run smack into the old program— fear of being found out, running away from forbidden feelings—but this was crazy. I was free now to have these feelings, to enjoy them . . . wasn't I? Sleep did not come. I tossed and turned, working through scenario after scenario in my mind. I would force myself to interact with this woman. She would reject me. I would persist. She would give in. We would become lovers. Wait! I didn't even know her and now I was having fantasies about having a relationship with her? Had I lost my mind? I felt as though I definitely had.

I awoke the next day feeling nervous about what lay ahead. On Sunday morning, the tall woman seemed quite relaxed, seemingly unbothered by my unconscionable behavior toward her. Maybe she hadn't noticed, maybe she didn't care. We proceeded through the day's activities, and I continued to avoid her. The workshop was scheduled to end at five o'clock. At four-thirty some urgent force within me asserted itself. I have to pay attention to this woman. I simply have to!

"Well, Terry," I said tentatively, "uh, I'd like to know what you're feeling."

She looked at me for a long moment before she spoke.

"I'm feeling avoided by you. I almost didn't come back, but I was curious to see what you would do today."

"I'm sorry. I have avoided you. That was wrong of me. I apologize."

"But, why? I don't understand it."

"I don't understand it either," I said honestly.

One of the men clapped his hands gleefully. "Oh, I wish we were starting all over again so you two could work this out!"

That prompted me to announce that the workshop was over and we would have some refreshments before we said good-bye. We sat in a circle, eating, drinking, and chatting. Terry moved over and sat next to me. I felt nervous with her so near me. I also felt excited. At one point, she gently put her arm around me. Reflexively, I laid my head on her shoulder, astonishing myself. We sat like that, without speaking, for what seemed like a long time. There was a kind of calming strength about her that felt comforting. At five o'clock, the group members began packing up to leave, and we said our good-byes. Only Terry and I were left in the room.

"Would you like to come home with me?" I blurted out. Oh no! Did those words really come out of my mouth?

"Sure," she said casually. "I'd love to."

Somewhere between Topanga Canyon and the Hollywood Hills, I panicked. I could see her car in my rearview mirror and it felt too close, too dangerous. What was I doing? I didn't know anything about this person. I'd better get away from her. I went barreling around corners, speeding up, turning down side streets, but she stayed with me. I couldn't believe it when she pulled up behind me in my driveway.

"That was a merry chase!" she laughed.

"Sorry, I forgot someone was following me," I lied.

Terry put her arm around me and once again I felt its calming effect. We

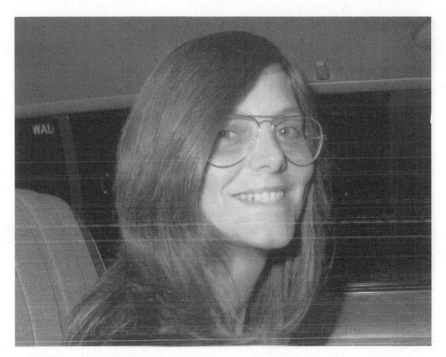

The woman I met in 1973 who seemed too young for me, but she persisted.
I have been with Terry ever since.

spent several hours talking. I don't remember who initiated our moving closer that night. I only remember that it felt good. She stayed the night and came back the next night and the next. Something began to solidify between us, but I didn't feel easy about it. I was disconcerted by the realization that I was clearly not in control of this situation.

In 1973 Terry DeCrescenzo worked as a counselor in a treatment facility for delinquent teenage girls. I learned that she came from an Italian Catholic, working-class family in East Boston and that they threw her out at seventeen when they learned she was gay. Compared to the rejected and homeless gay and lesbian kids Terry would later work with, she'd had a protected and nurturing childhood. She also had the discipline of a Catholic girls' school and the knowledge that she had been loved and cherished by her parents before they ran smack into the wall of their own inability to understand a daughter who seemed to stray so far from what they understood life to be about.

I had a hard time getting a handle on my feelings about Terry. One minute I felt as though I were in love with her, the next I was plotting how to end the relationship. It didn't help that she was seventeen years my junior and that we didn't seem to have much in common. I seized upon these to convince myself that this relationship was not going to work. I had endless conversations with myself:

"Terry is too young and inexperienced in the world for me. She's never even been on an airplane!"

"But, think about it. She's twenty-nine years old and owns a three-bedroom house, two cars, and a boat, all acquired on her own. She also has a savings account and a stock portfolio. A stock portfolio! Where were you at twenty-nine?"

I didn't want to think about where I was at twenty-nine, living in a tiny rented apartment with canvas chairs and a wooden telephone-cable spool for a table, just making it from paycheck to paycheck, not giving a thought to anything so grown up as a savings account, much less a stock portfolio. This internal dialogue went on for a long time.

At regular intervals I withdrew from Terry, but every time I pulled away, I missed her and came back. Incredibly she tolerated this yo-yo behavior. She was always there to take me back, which was flattering, compelling, and unnerving. I could feel myself becoming more dependent on her, needing her presence, but fearing something about that need that I didn't understand.

We went on for some time like that, spending most of our time together but living in separate houses. Having my own house gave me a feeling of independence, which seemed crucially important to me at the time. One thing was clear—having Terry in my life meant that being gay was no longer an abstraction. In my mid-forties the fact of being a lesbian was inescapable. It was no longer an open question, but a sexual and emotional reality. Activist slogans aside, this was ground zero for being gay.

It took a year of therapy to sort out my reasons for not allowing Terry completely into my heart. I had to core out my resistance to fully accepting my sexual identity, even when there seemed no ostensible reason to go on rejecting it, but little by little I was healing, giving myself permission to love and be loved.

Then there developed the looming threat that I might have pushed Terry away one too many times. I had gotten briefly involved with another woman and, for the first time, Terry did the same. I was filled with alarm, and I realized how much I cared about her and how much I needed her. I put on a concerted campaign to win her back. Reluctantly, she agreed to try again, though she remained wary of me for many months.

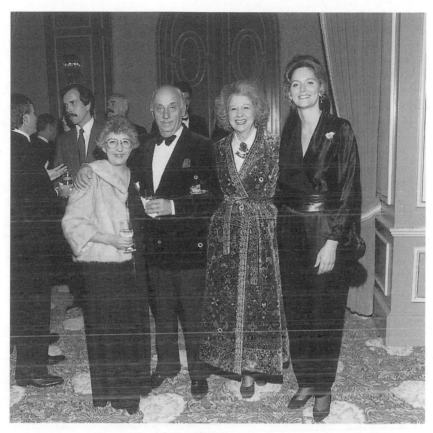

My family at a Gay and Lesbian Community Services Center dinner. With me are Dad, Trude (his sixth wife but the only one I ever considered my stepmother), and Terry, by then the president of the GLCSC board. (Courtesy of Barry Levine)

Eventually it worked, we were joined in Holy Real Estate in a wonderful big house that continues to be our home to this day. I began to feel for the first time that I was no longer the wanderer of my dream. I realized this relationship with Terry was the best thing that ever happened to me—the closest, deepest, and most loving connection with another human being I'd ever experienced. Her patience with my ambivalence, her ability to love me no matter how I behaved, her understanding of my struggle to come fully to terms with being a lesbian, were gifts I finally came to my senses enough to cherish. And I was seeing more clearly all the time what an extraordinarily talented individual she was in her own right.

In the mid-1970s, Terry earned a master's degree in social work at the

University of Southern California and began to branch out in her professional life. It started to feel more like we were peers. She also developed a warm relationship with my family. My mother thought she was the perfect daughter, and my father introduced her to people as his daughter-in-law. My stepmother Trude (the last and best of the six Mrs. Berzons) confided in her like a friend. She charmed my sister, niece, nephews, aunts, uncles, and cousins. Little by little, she infiltrated my life until it felt like something was wrong when she wasn't around.

Far from the unworldly innocent I had tried to reject in the early years of our relationship, Terry through the years has become a powerhouse. Tough, accomplished, and savvy, she has grown to be a major player in her profession and in the gay and lesbian community. I have proudly watched ceremonies in which she was honored as California Social Worker of the Year and Distinguished Alumnus of the Year at the University of Southern California School of Social Work. In 1980, Governor Brown appointed Terry to the California Board of Behavioral Science Examiners, the official watchdog agency for social workers, educational psychologists, and marriage and family therapists in the state. She was the chairperson of that important body for two years. In 1982 she became the first woman president of the Board of Directors of the Gay and Lesbian Community Services Center.

One day Terry came to me and asked, "What do you think about an agency to provide homes and services for gay and lesbian teenagers who are homeless—Gay and Lesbian Adolescent Social Services?"

"Sounds daring. Who is going to do that?"

"I am."

And in 1985, starting with a bank loan, unyielding optimism, and a defiance of the homophobic proscriptions that had kept anyone from doing this in the past, Terry started GLASS. She had always been interested in the problems of young people, having worked fourteen years with teenage delinquents. Adolescence is a particularly troubled time for those who are gay or lesbian. When these young people are estranged from family or have no viable family, it is not uncommon for them to live out their alienation on the streets, caught in the self-destructive cycle of drugs, alcohol, and prostitution. These are the "high-risk" kids who become residents of the GLASS houses and the recipients of that agency's services.

Many of the GLASS graduates, formerly street kids, have achieved a young adulthood in which they go to college or work and have plans for a future free of the destructive behavior that brought them to the agency. The foster-family project of GLASS matches infants, children, and teens with gay and lesbian foster families and currently has over one hundred children in placement. I see close-up now how Terry perseveres in everything she does, how confident she is about what can be accomplished, how loyal she is to the people she cares about. She is a tireless and shameless fundraiser for her kids and as good an example as there is of someone who has turned being "different" into a force for making a difference.

After twenty-nine years together I am more enamored and in awe of her than ever. She has made my life richer and more fun and created the opportunity for me to do what I've always wanted to do—write books. I shudder to think how I might have lost that car in the rearview mirror, running from myself, escaping what seemed too close, too fast, and too dangerous, only to find out that I was wrong about all of those things.

During the 1970s, the progress made by the gay rights movement also illuminated just how far there was yet to go. The antigay discrimination that had been taken for granted for so long began to feel odious, unacceptable, a challenge impossible to turn away from. Although only a small portion of the gay and lesbian population involved themselves at first, with each passing year more people came out of the closet and into the movement, motivated by a growing awareness of the outrageousness of societal attitudes against gays—hostility in the workplace, police brutality, street violence, public humiliation, and abuse in the courts.

Gay and lesbian people are not, historically, fighters. We are a gentle, caring people. We work in the helping professions, love to love, are caretakers and creators of beauty. What helped to blast us out of our passivity was the rage of the rioters at Stonewall, the fury of gays stunned at the lenient sentence of Dan White, Harvey Milk's assassin, and the angry protests of ACT UP at the failure of our government to adequately address the exploding AIDS crisis. Rage meant waking up to the pernicious campaigns to erode the freedoms of gay and lesbian people waged by the powerful religious right. Rage meant getting serious about fighting back.

During the 1970s I immersed myself in this movement for gay rights. It was exciting—playing the edge, inventing a new reality, feeling the comradeship of others equally zealous about what we were doing. As increasing numbers of people began to come out of the closet and get involved, they brought with them organizational skills, professional expertise, financial resources, and new energy to the movement. Unfortunately, some also brought radical political agendas, gender antagonisms, and hostility born of their own failed dreams.

The mix was volatile and, not surprisingly, exploded into a crisis in 1975 that threatened the very existence of the Gay Community Services Center. This story will sound familiar to anyone who has been involved in a nascent social movement.

Early evening, April 24, 1975, I received a frantic call from Morris Kight.

"My dear, you must come down here immediately! Drop everything. This is an emergency!"

Morris was given to drama, but the urgency in his voice convinced me of the sincerity of his concern. The Center was in the middle of moving from the old Victorian on Wilshire to a larger, newer building on Highland Avenue. I arrived at the old Victorian to find a confrontation going on between twenty or so scowling dissidents and several nervous-looking board members. The scene was in progress in a room bare of furniture except for a single chair on which Sheldon Andelson sat, his two elegant whippets, Pussy and Willy, posing on either side of him. Across the room the dissidents stood, arms folded, staring at the board members. The incongruity of the flannel-shirted, sandaled, angry young men and women facing down Sheldon and his whippets was almost comical, but the performance that followed was anything but amusing.

The group's spokesperson was Brenda, who in a scene right out of the Alfred Dreyfuss trial shot out her accusations, stabbing the air with her finger to punctuate each item of the indictment. "*J'accuse! J'accuse!*" I sat on the floor and listened while I was accused of misappropriation of government funds, mismanagement of Center projects, and criminal malfeasance. Brenda wrapped up her diatribe with a ringing demand for the immediate resignation of the entire board. The dissidents thrust their fists into the air and roared their approval.

The board members sat in shocked silence. The whole thing felt surreal. Here we were, individuals who had busted our asses to make this Center the best it could be and now we were being attacked for it by our own people. It made no sense. I was stunned. Sheldon broke the silence by asking several questions of the dissidents. Questions didn't seem to fit into their plan because suddenly they put their heads together, conferred, and quickly left the room without a word. Puzzled, Sheldon asked, "What happened?" Morris, more experienced in these matters, answered, "I think they've gone to caucus."

Whatever they went to do, they never came back, leaving us more perplexed and confused than ever. Was it over? Not by a long shot. It was only the beginning. We soon learned that these dissidents had contacted all of the Center's funding agencies, local, state, and federal, telling them that the GCSC was in crisis and unable to continue delivering funded services. The board immediately began damage control and a six-day marathon meeting to find out what was really going on. An investigation documented that there had been no misappropriation of funds and that the entire eruption was initiated by eleven people, some disaffected employees, some whose motivation is still a mystery.

The board met every night and all weekend, mainly to react to each day's actions by the dissidents. The board at that point consisted of Morris, Sheldon, a young psychiatrist named Ben Teller, and me, the other members having opted out of the conflict. One night I was feeling really fed up with the antics of the dissidents.

"Let's just fire them! We know who the eleven troublemakers are. Let's fire them right now!"

Others argued with me, but I persisted, having no idea what I was doing and no perspective on the agonies or remedies of social movement organizations. I was simply acting out of resentment, unaware that I was inviting the ax to fall, giving the dissidents exactly what they needed to escalate their action.

The next day the eleven were fired, and the entire Center staff then went on strike, joined by members of the community recruited with assaultive propaganda about the evil board out to exploit vulnerable gays. They picketed the Center, shoving and spitting on anyone who tried to enter. They telephoned death threats to the board. It got very ugly, culminating one terrible night in a siege that threatened to burn the building down and the board members with it.

We were meeting in a first-floor conference room at the back of the new Center building on Highland. Suddenly, the strikers were marching outside chanting wildly:

"CLOSE IT DOWN OR WE'LL BURN IT DOWN! BURN IT DOWN! BURN IT DOWN!"

The strikers' fury escalated. The noise was so great we had to shout to be heard inside the room. They began pounding on the windows. I looked up to see in the window the face of a beautiful young woman contorted in anger, her features frozen in an Edvard Munchian cry of outrage. She was one of my group trainees and a friend. What insanity was this? Friend against friend? How gullible people can be, allowing themselves to be misled into villain-victim scenarios, manipulated into violent protest with little or no real evidence that a wrong has been done to them.

The face at the window disappeared and a few minutes later we heard the strikers inside the building. One of the board members leaped out of his chair and began pushing a table against the door. We all began piling chairs on top of the table. I had participated hesitantly at first, thinking this was an overly dramatic reaction, but my hesitancy disappeared when I heard the bodies ramming against the outside of the door.

What were they thinking of doing when they got inside the room? We all pushed against the table. The door held, and after twenty nerve-wracking minutes, the strikers seemed spent. Gradually they withdrew and were gone. If they meant to scare us silly, they had certainly succeeded. I was shaking and didn't feel safe until I had been escorted to my car and was speeding toward home.

After our night under siege, the board held all its meetings in Sheldon Andelson's law offices (Pussy and Willy ever present). The board met far into each night for weeks, determined to get to the reasons for the upheaval. Rumors abounded: Were *agents provocateur* fomenting dissent as a way of neutralizing the growing visibility of the gay rights movement? It was said that the FBI had been known to use such tactics in the past to unsettle minority civil rights organizations. Or was this just the "circular firing squad," the phenomenon that sometimes plagues social reform movements when the anger meant for external targets is turned inward out of frustration.

Eventually, the real story came out. The precipitating cause of the agitation was that the women workers of the center felt marginalized within their own community (later, members of racial and ethnic minorities would begin to protest the same issues). These Center women did not trust the men who dominated the organization and consequently believed the men might turn the sizable government grant that had been awarded for women's alcoholism services to their own advantage. As a consequence of the disruption caused by the strike, the women did end up with funding for the free-standing Alcoholism Center for Women, which exists to this day, providing many years of excellent service to its clients. I deeply regret, however, that so many goodhearted, well-intentioned people on both sides had to suffer so much anguish. The strike continued for months, the violence finally ending as the action progressed to a lawsuit that went on for years.

The GCSC strike was a painful experience for me, but I learned a valuable lesson from it. In years to come I would personally work hard to ensure that every organization I had anything to do with had cosexual leadership and a true sharing of decision-making authority by men and women. It has always been my strong belief that an essential element in the progress of our community is gay men and lesbians working closely together, respecting one another's differences but drawing strength from what we have in common.

I became more savvy about a lot of things as a result of the trouble at the Center. In subsequent years I would see people who had been bitter enemies during the strike working together, socializing with ease, and resuming their friendships. At first I was puzzled, but I soon realized that this is one of the survival lessons one learns in a social movement and in politics generally. Yesterday's adversary may be tomorrow's ally. Political movements have their own forward momentum. One moves with the change or gets left in the dust.

When the strike was over and the rebuilding begun, I resigned from the board, exhausted and burned out, but I did continue to train group leaders and consult on Center programs. At that time, Terry began a ten-year stint on the Center's Board of Directors, three of them as its president.

By the beginning of 1976, I had recovered from my burnout and was ready to get into the action again. I joined the board of the San Francisco–based Whitman-Radclyffe Foundation, whose mission was to educate the public about homosexuality. I was impressed by their full-page ad campaign of the year before featuring a photograph of diverse people emerging from a closet: "Ten million Americans live in a closet. You would never suspect their curious habitat because they are your teacher, your plumber, your football hero, your best friends. And, yes, perhaps your son or daughter, your father or mother, or you." That ad appeared in *Time, Newsweek,* the *Wall Street Journal,* and *Harper's,* among other publications. Pretty heady stuff for 1975.

At Whitman-Radclyffe I took on the task of compiling a series of pamphlets built around important issues in gay and lesbian life. I recruited authors and formed an editorial board. This project became a major part of Whitman-Radclyffe's public information campaign and demanded a significant commitment of time on my part.

My other main activity with Whitman-Radclyffe was the formation of a Southern California women's support group for the foundation (there was already a men's group). No activist organization that I knew of existed for middle-class lesbians. The new group could be a social outlet for women who did not have the easily accessible gathering places that gay men enjoyed, a place where women could meet other lesbians like themselves. The group could also develop consciousness-raising activities to bring them more into the gay movement and offer personal-growth programs to help them feel better about themselves. The foundation would provide the initial financial support, and the women's group, in turn, would eventually contribute (financially and otherwise) to the other programs of the foundation.

I had a very personal reason for forming this women's group. I had spent so many years resisting positive feelings toward women. Now I wanted to work through this resistance. I saw Southern California Women for Whitman-Radclyffe as a way for me to open the door to other lesbians in my life.

Starting an organization was easy for me. I worked it all out on paper first, as I do with many things. Once I got the steering committee formed and functioning I thought it was time to have an election. I sincerely put out that I wasn't a candidate for any of the offices. I had only wanted to start the group and to be a part of it. We held the election and I counted the votes. Terry was elected chair. I was afraid that was indirectly a vote for me, so (with Terry's permission) I switched the results and announced that a woman who was an old friend of mine had been elected chair. That was my first mistake.

What I hadn't anticipated was that everyone would keep looking to me as the leader, and my old friend, not the secure and mature person I thought she was, would grow resentful. I took her out to dinner to talk about it. She assured me that she didn't have these feelings, but almost immediately she started a stealth campaign to squeeze Terry and me out of the organization. I had no idea what was going on until strange things began to happen. Terry and I would arrive at meetings only to find a locked door or an empty room. Finally, a member of the steering committee came to me with the truth about what was happening.

I learned that "move the meeting" was a tactic used to drive a targeted person out of an organization. I felt blindsided, stunned, bewildered. I was hurt that my friend would do this to me, angry at myself for being so naive. I didn't know what to think about the other women on the steering committee, but one thing was sure: I'd tried to open the door to lesbians in my life and it felt as though the door had been slammed in my face.

Shortly after that I resigned from the board of the Whitman-Radclyffe Foundation. I took the pamphlet series, its authors, and my editorial board with me and continued to work on the project until it became a book, *Positively Gay*, published in 1979, revised and updated in 1992 and in 2001. I'm glad to say that the organization I started, now called Southern California Women for Understanding, still exists, providing just the kinds of resources and activities I had originally intended. With the threat of my presence gone, my slippery friend did a good job of building an organization that continues to serve the needs of middle-class lesbians in Southern California.

Along with the excitement and travails of my activist life, I was faced in the early 1970s with the challenge of earning a living. When Bell & Howell suffered reverses that wiped out my easy job, I started an urban growth center in Los Angeles doing workshops and seminars, but that was strictly soft money. In an effort to stave off poverty, I took on several projects that were far afield from my activist interests. The first was the design and production of a training video to strengthen the motivation of grade-school students to achieve in school. I produced *McKeever the Achiever* at the UCLA Media Center. The project was funded by a nonprofit subsidiary of the U.S. Department of Education. They liked *McKeever* so much that we went on to develop a multimedia program to teach elementary school children something about emotions. I was drawn to this challenge because I had thought for a long time that a serious flaw in our education system was the total absence of any curriculum on the two things that every human being has to cope with throughout life, feelings and relationships.

The program itself was a series of ten-minute dramatized stories on audiotape, each followed by ten minutes of interactive exercises that the children did in groups of six. The storyline involved the Jack of Hearts who lived with his parents, the Queen and King of Hearts. Even with all the advantages Jack enjoyed, something very important was missing in his life. He didn't know what it was, but he knew that he would have to leave the familiar and comfortable surroundings of the Royal Kingdom to solve the mystery of his incompleteness. Jack's travels took him to the land of the Feelings, where he met the Sads, the Glads, the Mads, the Happys, the Hurts, and the Scareds, who taught him what they were all about and agreed to return to the Royal Kingdom and become part of his life.

The Heart Smart Adventures featured original music, sound effects, colorful visuals, and a complex storyline. The dramatizations on audiotape were performed by professional actors. Without particularly meaning to, I had produced a metaphorical tale that reflected my own journey of self-discovery. For me, something had been "not right" a long time, and I too eventually had to "leave home" to find what was missing in my life. Like Jack, I found it, and I think it was in celebration of that fact that I wrote *The Heart Smart Adventures* as I did.

We tested *Heart Smart* in many schools in the Los Angeles Unified School District over a period of four years. The children loved the program, as did the teachers. When the project was over, I shipped the finished product along with volumes of research data on its effectiveness to the funding agency. I waited to hear that the program was being used in schools all over the country as planned, but it made it only to a few schools in Pennsylvania and Delaware. Four years of my time, a quarter million dollars of the government's money, and the efforts of dozens of talented people, all virtually for nothing.

It wasn't the first time, and it certainly wouldn't be the last time, the U.S. government wasted taxpayers' dollars. I have tried to retrieve the program for people who know of it and want to turn it into a children's television series, but I developed it on salary, and thus it belongs to the U.S. government. I would never again make such a mistake with a creative product. The saving grace for me was that this project supplied me with the time, the facilities, and the support services to do important work for the gay and lesbian community, and I do thank the taxpayers for that.

When the four-year *Heart Smart Adventures* project was officially over, I was once again faced with finding a way to earn a living. I was sure I couldn't expect any more federal grants if the focus of my work were to be improving the lives of homosexuals. I made a few inquiries of people I knew in the Washington funding agencies anyway, and the gist of their responses was "forget it." So, I rented an office with my old friend from the Center strike, Dr. Ben Teller, and I started a psychotherapy practice specializing in working with gay and lesbian clients.

One day in late 1976, Ben asked me if a friend of his could use our group therapy room for the first meeting of an organization he was starting for gay academics and professionals. I liked that idea, and on December 5, people crowded into our suite to hear a young professor of English named Jay Hayes propose the Western Gay Academic Union. Jay talked about how gay academics, graduate students, writers, artists, and professionals needed to have a way of overcoming the isolation we typically felt working in the heterosexual

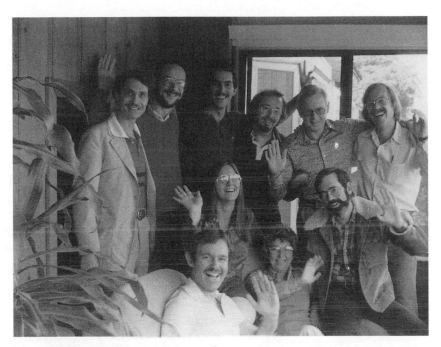

The founding steering committee of the Los Angeles Gay Academic Union in 1978.
Seated left to right: Don Carufo, Terry, me, and Ben Teller. Standing left to right:
John Alan Cohan, Sal Licata, Mark Hickey, Larry Lyon, Bob Hodges,
and Gary Steele.

world. He said we needed to help one another bridge the gap between our
gayness and our professional lives. The discussion was lively and intelligent.
I knew immediately that I was going to have a good time with this group.

Shortly after Jay's meeting, I was in New York and I met with the Gay
Academic Union people there. The GAU had started with seven men and
women in 1973, and by 1976 their annual conferences were attracting a thousand participants. The New York people had plenty of practical advice for
me: include students, they do the work and they have access to facilities for
conferences. Beware of people with radical political agendas. Recruit and
publicize, there's strength in numbers. They advised having male and female
cochairs, a surprising recommendation coming from New York, where the
gay movement, until AIDS, was overwhelmingly separatist.

Back in Los Angeles, a dedicated group, six men plus Terry and me, became the steering committee of the WGAU. I became the cochair, and we
were off and running with monthly meetings, speakers, concerts, confer-

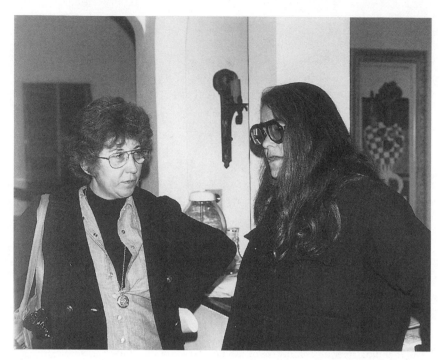

With Kate Millett at a GAU national conference, where she was the keynote speaker.

ences, and several publications. Jay Hayes, who had already lost an arm to cancer when he started the group, continued to work actively with the WGAU until the day he died in October 1979. A superb young man lost to us.

The Western Gay Academic Union was so successful that in January 1978 we became part of the national Gay Academic Union, whose headquarters moved to Los Angeles when I was elected its national president. The next two years were a whirlwind of activity for me. I traveled around the United States starting fifteen new GAU chapters. We established the GAU National Gay Research Network, publishing notices of studies in progress all over the country in our national newsletter. Through our scholarship fund, gay and lesbian students received awards that in some cases enabled completion of their education. Our national conferences were three-day affairs on university campuses wrapped up with gala banquets at which we presented awards to people such as Christopher Isherwood, Abigail Van Buren, and Governor Jerry Brown.

I even took the plunge again and started a women's group that was very much part of the WGAU but also met separately once a month. I had wised up by then and remained the unambiguous leader of the group. Many lesbian professionals and academics attended the monthly cultural events. I was slowly moving closer to women, making friends, developing working relationships, but always with some reserve, the old wariness unfortunately never far from the surface for me.

My strengths were in planning, designing, and organizing. Another psychologist, Rex Reece, and I started the Gay and Lesbian Mental Health Association, putting on programs for Los Angeles therapists interested in discussing psychological issues relevant to the lives of gay men and lesbians.

The salient event of 1979 for me was the publication of *Positively Gay*, and it was in relation to this that I had the most disturbing experience of the year. I had sent galleys of the book to Dick Farson, the former director of the Western Behavioral Sciences Institute and my mentor throughout the 1960s. My hope was that he would provide a blurb for the back cover. I also wanted him to be proud of me.

Dick had met Terry and had been quite cordial to us on a trip we'd made to visit him once so he knew by then that I was gay. I was therefore quite stunned when I received a letter from him saying that he couldn't endorse a book that "glorified" gayness. He wrote that presenting a list of eminent people who were gay to justify homosexuality was the same as offering a list of people who practiced incest or sadism or advocated slavery or believed the world was flat. He rejected the whole notion of gay advocacy as "absurd." I could not believe that this supposedly enlightened man, this "visionary thinker," this political liberal, would write such unenlightened, backward-thinking, reactionary drivel. I read the letter over and over, trying to find in it some saving grace, but there was none. I was furious with Dick and his arrogance in demeaning me and the work I had done. My response shot out of me. It took about three minutes to write.

> Dear Dick:
> I am deeply disappointed in you. Your bigotry doesn't bother me as much as your blindness to your own homophobia and hypocrisy. Your shallow thinking about "justifying homosexuality" and "glorifying gayness" is worthy of a fundamentalist, anti-life mentality, not of a supposedly enlightened, sophisticated humanistic psychologist and teacher.
> I am shocked at your unabashed equating of my orientation to lov-

ing another human being with the practices of "sadism," "incest," and "slavery." You would allow "rights of citizenship" (thanks) but "prideful excesses," is that really necessary? (Do you people really have to feel good about yourselves?)

Yes, you bastard, we do! Just as you do with your arrogant assertions about the non-acceptability of anything that doesn't reinforce your own narrowly defined and repressive view of human sexuality.

You bet you haven't been successful at "finding your way through these issues." I suggest you start with the terror of your own homosexual feelings that comes clearly through the thinly veiled hysteria of your comments. It is easy to see why externally imposed sexual taboos are so important to you.

Until I hear something to indicate that your homophobic white liberalism has been replaced with a real appreciation of what being gay is all about I shall consider it my responsibility to caution gay people struggling toward self-acceptance and self-esteem to steer clear of you.

His response was to thank me for my "penetrating insights" into his personality.

I have never seen nor heard from Dick Farson since. From time to time my nongay La Jolla friends try to get me to reconcile my relationship with Dick. I explain over and over that there was once a person in my life named Dick Farson, whom I admired and loved and who was very important to me. That person no longer exists.

What causes love to turn to rage? Usually it's betrayal. In this case, Dick betrayed my belief in him as an enlightened, compassionate person. The betrayal shook me up, called into question whatever confidence I had in my ability to accurately assess the values of the people close to me. It has been a very long road from self-alienation to the gay advocacy that defines much of what I do with my life now. Dick Farson calls that advocacy "absurd." The rage I feel about that is what every gay or lesbian person feels, or should feel, when betrayed by some nongay person they love and value. Our strength is in our refusal to be trivialized. Our power is in using our anger to expose the betrayal.

∝∾ 16

By the end of 1979 I was beginning to feel the effects of too much activity. I was constantly in motion, planning, talking on the phone, conducting meetings, attending fundraisers, recruiting money/people/ resources. I had begun to feel estranged from myself and resentful that I had so little time for a personal life—a sure sign of burnout. Though Terry worked right alongside me in all these projects, our relationship suffered from too little personal time alone together. By December it was apparent to me that I needed to pull back, so I phased out of my leadership role in the GAU.

I liked having more time to myself, but I also felt a little disoriented, no phones ringing, no meetings, no crises. Maybe I pulled back too fast. Divers come up slowly from the deep. I'd emerged precipitously. A part of me began to feel too isolated, too lost to the action, bored and useless. Instead of enjoying my quieter life, I was resenting it. Activist angst set in. There must be something I could be doing.

As if on cue, in May 1980, I got a call from Don Clark, urging me to come to the rescue of our mutual friend, Don Knutson, whose organization, Gay Rights Advocates, was going through a palace revolt. Don Knutson was an attorney, a constitutional law expert, and a law professor who taught for many years at the University of Southern California and Stanford. In 1977, Don Knutson was approached by a young law student, Richard Rouilard, with family wealth who wanted to fund a public-interest gay law firm to advance the civil rights of gays through precedent-setting litigation. Knutson accepted the offer and with Richard founded the San Francisco–based Gay Rights Advocates.

GRA successfully litigated cases dealing with child custody, recognition of gay student groups, employment discrimination, and gay-exclusionary policies of the Immigration and Naturalization Service. Part-time lawyers, work-study students from law schools, and cooperating attorneys from other law firms all became part of GRA. Maybe the organization grew too fast, for despite its success, or maybe because of it, a small group of young lawyers rebelled against Knutson's leadership and tried to oust him, the circular firing squad at work again.

I answered the alarm and joined the board of directors of GRA. It took almost a year, but the organization was salvaged, Knutson remained at the helm, and GRA became National Gay Rights Advocates, continuing to litigate landmark cases. I originally agreed to stay only until the trouble was over, but working with that superb group of people kept me on that board for four years. My old friend Knutson was a very dear, genteel, sophisticated, and charismatic companion. My new acquaintance, Richard Rouilard, was a brilliant, forward-thinking, uproariously funny young man who would become a close friend and a member of my gay family.

Throughout the more than twenty years I spent as a young adult in therapy with psychoanalytically oriented psychiatrists I was always assured by them that I was not really homosexual. The pronouncement resonated deep within me and set up the condition for a conflicted identity that plagued me for years to come. In 1980 I was presented with a glorious opportunity for rebuttal. I was invited to speak to the fourteenth annual meeting of the American Academy of Psychoanalysis on the topic "The Homosexual and Society."

On May 4, 1980, I stood before a packed ballroom and explained to the psychoanalysts gathered there that the only experience of "arrested development" I had suffered was the result of being encouraged by my therapists to live a lie for most of my adult life. I told of the despair I felt for being so flawed, the suicide attempts, the repression of feelings of affection toward women and how it had done irreparable damage to my ability to love and trust women even though I was now free to do so.

I told this audience that I had eventually rescued myself from psychoanalytic dogma about the meaning of homosexuality and found personal validation in my involvement with the liberated gay and lesbian community. I then talked about all the rich resources that our community offered for the affirmation of a positive gay identity and the evolution of mentally healthy gay and lesbian individuals unburdened by the need to distort their reality in order to feel "normal."

Although they listened politely and attentively, I had no way of knowing whether my message was getting through. Yet by giving that speech I passed a marker in my life—a point beyond which I was free of these advocates of denial who so diligently tried to "straighten me out." By standing before this audience and embracing the authenticity of who and what I was, I had truly moved beyond their reach at last.

In 1982, Terry and I had put our lives together in the serious way that buying a house represents. I spent the next few years in domestic tranquility, savoring the relationship that was increasingly at the center of my life. I came to realize how much I had learned about partnership from this woman seventeen years my junior but so much more mature than I in her understanding of how intimate relationships work and what it means to be family. We were busy integrating our books, our music, our dishes, and our furniture. That was the easy part. Much more difficult was the integration of our styles and interests because Terry and I are two people different in practically every way: family background, cultural experience, orientation to socializing, recreational interests, inclination to risk, concern about money, and level of comfort with the curveballs life throws us all. She tends to take everything in stride and wonders what I get so excited about. I tend to react, often with intensity, and wonder why she doesn't comprehend what a crisis we are in.

In the process of working out a life we can both live with, we have built compatibility, struggled to understand and embrace change, and appreciated and valued the ways in which we differ. We don't compete for the attention of our audiences, at least not usually, and we allow each other our idiosyncrasies, at least most of the time. I have learned a great deal about compromise, negotiation, and the many paths to conflict resolution.

Impressed with how successfully Terry and I have negotiated the rocky relationship road, I began working a lot with groups of same-sex couples, and soon I saw the commonalities that nearly all gay and lesbian couples have to deal with. In 1985 I started to write *Permanent Partners: Building Gay and Lesbian Relationships That Last*, which was published in 1988 by E. P. Dutton. It has been in print ever since, a bestseller on gay lists for years, and continues to sell steadily.

A key concept in *Permanent Partners* is the importance of assuming that one's relationship is permanent—no running away from problems; no retreating into silence, no escaping into drugs, alcohol, or outside sex, no moving on to the next lover. I came to see with Terry and through the work with my clients that the assumption of permanence enables partners to address the deeper underlying issues between them and to achieve the trust that makes real bondedness possible. Tempting as it is, flight doesn't work to solve problems. What works is sticking it out through the painful discussions until you understand what is really happening and what part you might have played in it. What works is allowing vulnerability, being able to admit you're wrong, and the willingness to change.

As I have traveled the country giving lectures and doing workshops on relationships since the publication of *Permanent Partners,* I have become increasingly convinced that these lessons are essential for gay and lesbian couples who have too often internalized the messages of society about our partnerships: can't work, won't last, don't count. Our relationships can work and last, and they absolutely do count just as much as we want them to. How dare straight society demean that which is so precious to so many of our people? How dare they decide for us how legitimate our loving relationships can be, what benefits we are entitled to, what religious or civil ceremonies should be available to sanction our partnerships? Why aren't we angrier about this?

I wonder why more gay and lesbian people aren't outraged at the arrogant moralists in Congress and state legislatures who vote against our right to marry as though we are not equal enough to them to deserve that privilege? Of course, some in our community are not advocates of gay marriage, which is fine. The issue here is choice, the opportunity to be able to marry if that is what one chooses. An example of the absurdity of the moralists' stand is Richard Ramirez, the California serial killer who raped and murdered thirteen women. He was allowed while on death row to legally marry the person of his choice because his sexual orientation was correct. Why is it that a convicted serial murderer can marry and a decent, law-abiding gay or lesbian citizen cannot? Why aren't we outraged?

The C. C. Construction Company in Palm Springs is a gay disco with the usual ear-splitting music and jam-packed dance floor. The Board of National Gay Rights Advocates had just concluded a weekend retreat in 1981, and we were winding down to the beat of whatever was passing for music at the moment. Above the din, someone was shouting at me, "Have you heard about the new gay cancer?"

"The what?"

"Gay cancer. Six people have died of it so far."

"Gay cancer? What makes it gay?"

"All the people who died of it are gay men."

"I never heard of it."

"You will."

By 1983, over a thousand persons were known to be infected. Although the numbers of sick and dying continued to increase, HIV and AIDS were not yet big news in the country's media. The shift occurred in July 1985 with the revelation that Rock Hudson had AIDS and was near death. Television coverage of the popular actor's illness over the next four months became regular fare on the evening news. It would, however, take our president two more years to break what Randy Shilts called Ronald Reagan's "thunderous silence" on the subject of AIDS.

It was for Reagan's sins of omission that participants in the 1987 March on Washington for Lesbian and Gay Rights turned their faces to the White House as they strode past 1600 Pennsylvania Avenue to roar one word repeatedly: "Shame! Shame! Shame!" By then, twenty thousand Americans had died of AIDS, yet the president of our country was still virtually silent on the subject, as though it weren't happening at all.

The numbers of men and women affected by AIDS have been staggering. I have lost friends, colleagues, and clients to AIDS, and with every death my sadness has deepened. When I've thought I had no more tears, more came. I have cried for some of the people I've written about in this book—my dear friends, the cofounders of the National Gay Rights Advocates, Don Knutson and Richard Rouilard. Four of the six men with whom Terry and I founded the Gay Academic Union in Los Angeles. Rex Reece, Judge Rand Schrader, Fred Greene, who did the brilliant illustrations for *The Heart Smart Adventures*, and Jeff Beane, my research assistant on that project. Jim Foster, who looked into the camera at that 1972 Democratic Convention and told America, "I am a gay man." Freeman Pollard, Sheldon Andelson, and others too numerous to name here.

Sometimes, when I'm lying in bed at night or waiting in a bank line or driving the long stretches of Los Angeles freeways, my mind plays tricks. I think of calling a particular person about something, and the truth slams into my brain—"You can't call him, he's dead." I cannot fathom this person gone. It makes no sense—too young, too vibrant, too alive.

"How can he be gone?"

"What do you mean he's dead?"

Going to funerals and memorial services became common occurrences in the lives of gay and lesbian people in the 1980s and '90s. The biological families of those gay men who succumbed to AIDS were sometimes present at these commemorations, sometimes not, but the chosen gay and lesbian families of the person were always there. If one needed evidence of the substantive connection that our chosen gay families provide in our lives, one need look no further than memorial services for those who have died of AIDS.

Sometimes the biological family, carrying the denial of their "loved one's" homosexuality to his grave, held sanitized services from which the person's gay and lesbian friends were banned, at which no mention was made of gayness or AIDS. My inclination to pity these families for the agony they inflicted upon themselves is matched only by my anger at them for the pain they added to the grief of people who probably knew their child better and loved him more completely than these families of origin ever did.

We have delivered our eulogies, held one another and cried, committed to carry in our minds forever the memory of our dear friends. There is so much to be learned from the extraordinary caring that many gay and lesbian people have come to experience through the periods of nursing our friends and the times of grieving together. We have soothed and comforted those we loved as they were dying and helped them take leave of us with all the dignity that was their due. We have carefully composed our eulogies to make sure there is recorded in the hearts of all those present the significance of each and every life.

Being a therapist to gay men in the 1990s has involved doing things that psychotherapists don't usually find themselves doing. When my clients with AIDS became too weak to come to my office, I went to their homes. When they became too sick to be at home, I went to the hospital. I've touched my face to their gaunt, unshaven faces. I have silently said good-bye to them during such moments, and when they died, I went to their funerals and memorial services.

I feel on friendlier terms with death now than I did before all this started. It still frightens me, but death is no longer the menacing stranger it used to be. I have watched vigorous young men take leave of their lives slowly, regretfully, sometimes fighting all the way, but more often calmly accepting death as the release from pain that it is. I have measured my own courage against that of the people with AIDS I have known. I have seen where I am wanting, where I must come to terms with fear more effectively if I am to face whatever the future holds with the grace that these people have shown in their dying. And there have been lessons about living from these people with AIDS—living with debilitating illness, pain, the uncertainty of what's coming next, but living with all this defiantly, culling every moment of gaiety, adventure, humor, and human connectedness from whatever life is left to them.

From the caretakers of those suffering with AIDS I have also learned volumes about compassion and the ability to be selfless in the face of another's need. I have seen men and women transcend their own expectations of what they were capable of and what they could tolerate as the physical and emotional demands of caring for a person with AIDS escalated beyond anything they could have imagined.

There is a new kinship now among men and women who are gay, evolved in the shadow of death. This kinship is a vital force in the relationships of those who have shared a vigil for someone they loved. It has been a potent experience to witness the playing out of the AIDS drama, a lesson in the power of love and the strength of the human spirit. If there is anything positive to come out of this terrible tragedy, surely it is the new awareness that we gay and lesbian people have of ourselves as a strong, resilient, deeply caring community capable of meeting staggering responsibilities. This, I believe, is the legacy of AIDS.

There was a bit of a chill in the air that Wednesday evening in 1986, cool for the month of May in Los Angeles. Terry and I were sitting outside talking about the day. I crossed my arms against my chest to warm myself, and as my left hand brushed across my right breast, I felt something there. No, it was just my imagination. I tried to put the thought out of my mind, but my fingers wanted to return to the spot to feel it again. I excused myself and went into the bathroom where I examined my breast carefully. There was definitely a lump there.

I stayed alone in the bathroom for a few minutes, thinking about what to do. I had an appointment for a checkup the following month. Should I see a doctor sooner? I remembered the fuss about the lump I'd had years before—cancel my tour, get into the hospital right away—I'd ignored that and the lump turned out to be benign. All lumps are not malignant. This could be nothing. My mind began to fog over. I went back outside and said nothing to Terry about what I'd found.

When I called the doctor's office the next day, the chirpy receptionist said the doctor couldn't see me until Monday. I didn't mention the lump. It seems crazy now to have waited five days, but I wanted to believe there was nothing to worry about, so what difference would five days make?

In the gynecologist's office on Monday morning the doctor examined my breast and said he wanted an immediate mammogram. He told me not to worry, but the urgency in his voice when he called from the examining room to order the mammogram was anything but reassuring. I was beginning to feel anxious. While the doctor was on the phone my mind reeled back to five months before, December, the last time I was in that room. In the middle of my examination, the doctor had been called out to deliver a baby. He never returned to examine my breasts. I wondered now, might he have detected this lump if he'd completed his exam then?

I liked my gynecologist. He was always reassuring when there was a problem. "Don't you worry about it. Let me do the worrying," he would say. Now the full force of that folly hit me. It was my body, my health, my life. Why was I so quick to abdicate responsibility, to let male physicians infantilize me as I had always done? I made a pact with myself to stay in control of my health care from then on. I left the gynecologist's office, and later in the day he called to say the mammogram was "inconclusive." He wanted me to see a surgeon right away.

I raced ahead of myself, panicked. A part of me had already decided it was cancer; I was ready, no surprises please. At that point I called Terry to tell her what was happening. On Tuesday we went to see the surgeon together.

There was an intensity about Dr. Stephen Shapiro that I liked. He did a needle biopsy, then sat with us in his office to explain what would happen if the biopsy showed cancer. He carefully and unhurriedly answered all our questions. I remember thinking what a patient and gentle man he was—for a surgeon. The next day we returned to Dr. Shapiro. He said he was sorry, but the biopsy was inconclusive. He recommended that I go into the hospital for a biopsy under anesthetic. If it was positive, they could perform the mastectomy immediately—one-stop surgery.

I decided I owed it to myself to get a second opinion. On Thursday, Terry and I visited another surgeon, who examined me, then told me to dress and come into his office. When Terry and I were seated in front of him, he turned to the shelves behind his desk and pulled out a large book. He opened it and placed it before us. "Now, I think reconstruction is very much in order. It can be done in several ways. Why don't you look at these pictures and see what appeals to you." With that he left the room.

Terry and I looked at one another. Slowly, absently, I turned a few pages, only glancing at the raw scars of before-and-after pictures of reconstructed breasts. I began to feel spaced-out, and I must have looked it. Terry gently took the book away from me and put it on the doctor's desk. "Let's get out of here," she said. We stood up to go. Just then the doctor returned. "See anything you like?" he asked. Not waiting for an answer, he said that we had to be concerned about the cancer having spread, so he'd ordered a series of tests for me and made the appointments. "Please sit down, and I'll explain where you go for these tests."

Without moving, I said, "I think I've missed something here. My biopsy was inconclusive, but from an examination you can tell that this tumor is malignant? And now we are moving right along to breast reconstruction?"

The doctor smiled, and spoke in a patronizing voice, "I'm sure you have cancer. Trust me."

The last thing in the world I wanted to do was to trust this man. My only thought was to get out of his office as quickly as possible. "I have to go home and think about all this," I stammered.

"Well, don't wait too long. Every day counts," he said ominously.

At this point I felt frightened and confused, but I wanted to make a sensible decision. I needed to talk to someone who understood all this. I thought of Peggy. Of course! I would ask her advice. Why hadn't I thought of it before? Everything had been happening so fast. How stupid of me. My friend Peggy Kemeny was a surgical oncologist!

Peggy was visiting in New York at the time, so I called and told her what was happening. She became quite agitated and asked, "How could you think of anyone but me doing this? This is what I do. I'll be back in Los Angeles on Sunday. I'll meet you at the City of Hope, eight o'clock Monday morning. Be there." And that was that.

Peggy did a biopsy under anesthetic. I waited in the small recovery cubicle for the results. When Peggy appeared, she had her hands jammed into the pockets of her hospital coat. She was already talking as she rounded the corner of the cubicle, as though she needed to get the words out as quickly as possible: "It is cancer." Terry was right behind her, looking quite pale. There is a moment when one hears such news in which everything comes to a complete standstill, time stops, the moment is preserved forever. The words hang in the air. "It is cancer."

When cognition resumed, my first thought was of how difficult it must be for my friend to be giving me this news. Then I thought of Terry and how hard this must be for her. I tried to reassure both of them that I was okay, but I couldn't hold back the tears. I cried from the most primitive part of myself where there are no defenses against the overwhelming dread of the unknown. Peggy suggested that I have the surgery in two days because there were tests to be performed first. I felt total trust in her. I knew she cared about me and would do her best for me.

The mastectomy took six hours, followed immediately by a procedure in which the plastic surgeon took tissue from my abdomen and made a new breast. The "transabdominal flap" left a twenty-four-inch scar running across my stomach from hip to hip. In the course of my "tummy tuck," they also removed abdominal muscles. What nobody told me was that recovery from this procedure would be excruciating. When I tried to stand and straighten up, the pain was searing. It went on for weeks.

At the insistence of the nurses, I dragged myself around the halls of the hospital bent in two, pleading with them to leave me alone. I only wanted to lay still in my pretzel-like misery, but they explained that I would be permanently like that if I didn't get up and walk around. It took a month of physical therapy and exercise after I left the hospital to strengthen the remaining abdominal muscles sufficiently to be able to bend and straighten in a normal fashion. Never mind. I had a new breast and a newly flat tummy. I'd had superb care from a loving friend. And I was alive.

Several weeks after I got home from the hospital, I had my first appointment with the oncologist who was going to follow my case. Dr. Michael Van Scoy-Mosher (he added his wife's name to his own) was slender and fine featured with a lot of curly brown hair and soft blue-gray eyes. His manner was warm and low key. I liked him from the beginning. Michael explained about the chemotherapy that I would receive every three weeks for the next six months. He said I could expect my hair to fall out, so I might want to buy several wigs as soon as possible. He said I would probably be quite sick from the treatments for about four days after each one, but that I would be okay to follow my usual routine the rest of the time. At the end of the discussion, Michael gently put his hand on my arm, smiling reassuringly as he did so, something he would always do at some point in every session, a moment of personal contact beyond the clinical.

The following week I started chemotherapy, and indeed my hair soon began to fall out, but by then I owned several quite fetching wigs. I lost every hair on my head and wore my wigs for a year. I had expected that losing my hair would be devastating, but it wasn't. I think having a totally supportive partner, who seemed unfazed by the changes in my appearance, helped me to accept all of those changes without trauma.

I was told that I was getting a very strong course of chemotherapy. I was plenty sick, but it wasn't as bad as I'd anticipated. Perhaps it was because I didn't fight it. I just accepted that I was going to feel rotten and be dysfunctional for four days every three weeks. I prepared myself for the worst and was relieved when the worst never came. During the first month of my recovery, though, I had some trouble sorting out the emotional side of what was happening to me. I learned that reading books about "battling cancer" made me feel depressed and frightened because they were full of information about the dire things that might lay ahead, so I stopped reading.

Michael referred me to a young psychiatrist who specialized in working with cancer patients. Terry and I saw him together a few times. He was very sweet and pleasant, but he had a tendency to explain life to me in a way that made me want to yell at him, "Give me a break! I was saying these things to people back in the '60s when you were in high school!" But I didn't. I liked him and didn't want to hurt his feelings. All in all, I found that returning to my routine, seeing clients, and resuming my writing constituted the best remedy for me. Within a few months, I seemed to stabilize emotionally.

When one contracts a life-threatening illness there is always a decision to make about whom to tell. Some people feel comfortable telling everyone. Others write books and appear on television talk shows. I applaud and admire that, but the thought of becoming a professional cancer patient was unappealing to me. I wanted my life to be as normal as possible. Of course I told family and our closest friends, but I did not tell my clients, although my clients who were physicians guessed the truth and called Terry to verify whether they had "gotten it all." It may seem strange for clients to be calling their therapist's spouse, but in the gay and lesbian community of Los Angeles, Terry and I were a highly visible couple and she was easily accessible to people. She simply could not lie to these doctors, so she told them the truth. None of them ever spoke to me about it, taking their cue from my silence on the subject, and I was glad. I wasn't ready to talk about it. I'm not exactly sure why I felt the need to be silent about my illness. Perhaps it tapped into the old program—I don't want to be different, I want to be like everybody else, I want to be normal. That little tune keeps playing somewhere inside me, and every now and then something happens to turn up the volume.

In the years since my surgery I have enjoyed good health, carefully monitored every six months by Michael Van Scoy-Mosher. Sometimes between checkups I have the experiences that every person who has had cancer goes through—lumps, bumps, and unexplained pains that trigger rushed visits to the doctor to check out any symptoms that are not immediately identifiable. There is always suspense while waiting for test results and great relief upon hearing that everything is okay. One tries to achieve détente with the anxiety that occurs each time an unexplained symptom appears. I have attempted to maintain a certain detachment during these times of uncertainty, but my unconscious is rarely fooled—as is apparent in the restlessness that replaces sleep and the preoccupation with nothing in particular that replaces the ability to concentrate.

One day I was in my oncologist's office talking to his nurse. I was saying something about an advance in AIDS treatment and how it was "a medical miracle." Michelle looked at me, "In this office we consider *you* a medical miracle." I can't imagine why, but I didn't question what she meant by that.

October 1996. Terry and I are having dinner with Peggy Kemeny who now lives in New York. She is talking about someone she knows who is having a rough time with a breast cancer diagnosis. Peggy uses me as an example of someone who had a worse case and is okay twelve years later.

"You're a medical miracle," she says.

I don't question her, but in the taxi going back to the hotel, I ask Terry, "What is this medical miracle business?" As we careen through the streets of Manhattan, Terry tells me the truth that she kept from me for twelve years.

"When Peggy came out of the operating room she told me that the cancer was worse than she'd thought. It was deep in the chest wall and she'd had to remove fifty-three lymph nodes that had cancer cells in them. I asked her what that meant and she said that you had maybe two years to live, maybe."

I sank back in the seat, stunned. "And you never told me this."

"No, I decided to keep it from you as long as I could. I forbade Peggy to tell you and she was very upset about it. She said that these days they always tell the patient the truth. I also forbade Michael to tell you."

"But this is twelve years later and I'm still alive. When did you stop expecting me to die?"

"About the third year after the surgery."

"And you carried this secret all that time? That must have been very tough to do."

"It was."

My brain is overloaded, in a state of shock. I have a very strong commitment to the truth, but I am also a person who tends to obsess. Was it better for me not to know that I was expected to die so soon? Would I have just given up and waited for the end? Probably, maybe, I don't know. But I do know that Terry took on an enormous responsibility. Did she have a right to do that? Was that courage or arrogance? What a burden to carry alone! My thoughts are jumbled, tumbling, I feel punchy. I had defied death and didn't even know it. That I didn't know seemed wrong, and yet so right. The rest of the cab ride is a blur.

Terry fretted that she shouldn't have told me at all.

"No. No," I protested, "it's best I know."

I'm still not sure. I'm working on it.

While having cancer felt earthshaking at the time, the postsurgical period had its moments of comic relief. Immediately upon my return from the hospital I had a private nurse who proved herself to be a menace. First she left a heating pad on my reconstructed breast, which of course had no sensation in it. By the time she realized what she'd done, my new breast was cooked and had to be treated with burn medication. Next, she forgot to hang onto my weakened frame as I was negotiating the stairs and I tumbled to the bottom, fortunately not breaking anything that wasn't already broken. Following the departure of Nurse Nemesis, we hired a woman from a nanny service. A nanny seemed just right, motherly, kind, and nurturing, but my nanny was none of those things. She was mean and bossy. When she decided that Terry reminded her of her own harsh and punishing mother, her "negative transference" sent her out the door.

Arnold came to us from a *Los Angeles Times* ad. He was a gentleman of indeterminate age with an impressive résumé, having worked as a cook/butler for the Shah of Iran, Baron Guy de Rothschild, and William and "Babe" Paley. He also adored dogs. By now we had not only elderly Raggy but two little Yorkie puppies, Minnie and Max. As we talked in the initial interview, Arnold cuddled our dogs, who all seemed to be mesmerized by him. He was overqualified for our modest household, but we hired him anyway.

Arnold was a gracious caretaker. He filled the house with flowers and made wonderful meals. It was only his sense of whimsy that gave me pause. Arnold loved the way our two little Yorkies tended to run side by side, like tiny horses prancing on parade. Once I caught him prancing with them, the drum major at the head of their formation. But sometimes Arnold would be displeased with Minnie and Max because of their resistance to being housebroken and their incessant barking at nothing in particular. "That's it! That's it!" he would scream. "It's Switzerland and the convent for you! The plane is leaving for Zurich and you're going to be on it!" Two perplexed puppies just gazed wide-eyed at Arnold. Old Raggy, protected from such carryings on by his inability to hear much of anything, turned his deaf ears to it all, put his head down, and went to sleep.

One day I came home to find Arnold in the kitchen cooking. The dogs were nowhere in sight.

"Arnold, where are the dogs?" I asked.

Without missing a beat, he answered, "The ladies are on the terrace sipping Calvados, smoking Turkish cigarettes, and reading French novels."

"And Raggy?"

"The gentleman is in the parlor having a cigar and brandy."

"I see. Thank you, Arnold."

In fact, the dogs were in the bedroom, hiding from a scolding, or was it one of Arnold's periodic demonstrations of smothering affection?

Following Arnold's departure from our household we decided to continue having help for a while because I was still not at full strength. We advertised and interviewed several dozen people. They came with their résumés and photograph albums and endless stories of the movie stars, directors, and producers they had worked for. To a person, they gossiped about these celebrity households, which we felt was alarmingly indiscreet even as we hung on their every word. After a while we began to feel like we were living in a Jackie Collins novel.

The coup de grâce was the former ballet dancer who had been sidelined by arthritis in his knees. The dancer's culinary skills were quite good, and we were satisfied with him until one day I came into the kitchen to find him sucking on a baby bottle. Startled, I asked him what he was doing. He said his nutritionist had put him on a diet of carrot juice designed to cure his arthritis, and he was supposed to drink it out of a baby bottle because the sucking would cause better absorption of the juice by his body. I was pretty sure I couldn't cope with a grown man sucking a baby bottle in my kitchen. So, feeling strong again, I decided I had had enough of helping hands. We reclaimed our kitchen and rejoiced at being alone in our own house again.

∝∾ 17

For gay people the defining event of 1987 was the National March on Washington for Lesbian and Gay Rights, half a million strong—exuberant college students with their university banners, middle-aged people, some looking as though they wondered how they got involved in all this, elderly gays and lesbians astonished to see such a happening in their lifetime, parents of gays, politicians, celebrities, every ethnic minority, age range, and socioeconomic strata. There were seasoned activists and people who had never in their lives participated in anything publicly gay. All marched under gray, overcast October skies, singing, shouting, chanting the rallying cries of gay pride.

Because I didn't think I could walk the distance, Freeman Pollard and I took the Metro and stationed ourselves at the rally site where we could see the marchers coming toward us, hundreds of thousands approaching over the horizon, wave after wave, until we were surrounded by them, the largest gathering of gay people ever in one place. It was almost unbearably moving to feel a part of this massive celebration, this explosion of energy.

At the front of the rally site there were rows of wheelchairs where people with AIDS sat quietly, a stark statement of what the protest aspect of this march was about. As the afternoon grew chilly, a call went out for blankets and sweaters for those in wheelchairs, and people took off their own sweaters to provide warmth for those sitting at the front. Soon a load of blankets arrived.

The march itself was the high point of a weekend of activity. On Saturday, two thousand gay and lesbian couples gathered on a blocked-off street in front of the IRS building to be "married" in a mass ceremony. Terry and I participated, exchanging rings and committing to the partnership that was already at the center of our lives. At sunrise on Sunday morning, the AIDS quilt was unfolded for the first time, two thousand panels the size of two football fields. The names of the dead were read aloud, each name read slowly and deliberately to emphasize the importance of each person as an individual. It was excruciatingly solemn and it went on for three hours.

On Monday, in an act of civil disobedience, hundreds of gay and lesbian people demonstrated on the steps of the United States Supreme Court Building. Six hundred who were arrested were prepared for this consequence by the training sessions they had attended on Saturday morning. All of the activities around the march were a thrilling affirmation of how potent people can become when mobilized to speak with one voice, channeling frustration and anger into a powerful experience of advocacy.

I left Washington profoundly moved, inspired to a new level of militancy in my activism. And I was not alone. Anguish about AIDS and anger at the Supreme Court's antigay ruling in a recent Georgia sodomy case raised the ire of an increasing number of gays who felt morally aggrieved and freed of the closet enough to begin a campaign of direct-action protests against the government and other establishment institutions. A transformation in consciousness was occurring in the gay and lesbian community.

I have written elsewhere about the bash that Terry and I put on to celebrate our fifteenth anniversary, but it was enough of a milestone event to bear repeating. First of all, we decided to go all out and host a black-tie dinner dance for one hundred and fifty of our closest friends at the fashionable Beverly Hills Hotel.

"Is this madness?" I wondered. "Would this swanky joint really go for a room full of faggots and dykes dancing and hugging and kissing and celebrating ourselves?" We'd been to dozens of gay community fundraisers at large hotels, but we'd never heard of anything publicly gay at the posh old pink palace on Sunset Boulevard. Just the kind of "first" Terry and I loved.

Our adventure began with the hotel catering manager, a woman of a certain age, steely gray eyes, blue hair, hauteur personified, she sat ramrod straight behind her rococo desk. Peering at us over gold-rimmed half-glasses, she smiled patronizingly and asked what we would like to arrange.

"A dinner dance," I said.

She daintily pulled a form out of the top drawer of her desk and began to write. "And is this event celebrating something?"

"Yes, a fifteenth anniversary."

She wrote. "And whose anniversary is this?"

"Ours."

She stopped writing, but she didn't look up. "Yours? The two of you?"

"Yes."

She did look up. We smiled. She nodded, looking off into the middle distance. "And when would you like to do this?"

"Sometime next month."

She pulled out a calendar and studied it. Finally, she suggested several dates. We picked one. She wrote. She then handed us menus and a price list. We could take them home, make our decisions, and let her know. She would mail us a contract. We said our good-byes and left.

Internalized homophobia lurks everlastingly in the nooks and crannies of even the most liberated gay or lesbian brain. I was absolutely certain we would receive not a contract but a letter from the Beverly Hills Hotel saying, they were sorry but . . . I was quite wrong. We received a contract and a polite letter saying they were happy to serve us and would look forward to our event. The world was changing. We were changing the world.

I spent the next few weeks in a studio editing a video that told the story of our fifteen-year partnership. We had still photos and film footage of us at home, giving parties, marching in parades, doing television interviews, giving speeches. I put it all together with a voice-over narrative and a music track, hardly Academy Award material, but a loving record of a life shared.

All our friends and members of our families attended the event. Everyone was formally attired, the men (and some of the women) in black tie, a handsome and exuberant crowd. At the end of the cocktail hour, a hush fell over the room as we announced we were going to take our vows of recommitment. We read in counterpoint the following:

As light comes to the day
And spring follows the retreat of winter
We illuminate each other's lives
And hold ourselves close for the warmth
That we create together.

We have traveled through many places in our journey
Not always venues to delight
There were the dark meanderings through tunnels
That seemed to have lost their openings
The terrible illusion of no exit
Until reason healed the sight
And there was light at both ends of the tunnel.

We've learned together and taught each other
We've forgotten the lessons and forsaken each other
But the road came around in a circle
And we were joined again, smarter, stronger,
And more bonded than before.

We know each other now
We've broken all the codes
And seen inside all the Chinese boxes
Inside Chinese boxes inside Chinese boxes.

We are an open book to one another
But we still turn the pages very carefully
Just in case a clue was overlooked, a nuance missed
A theme not fully comprehended.

Now we come before you
Our family who are friends
Our friends who are family
To renew a commitment to our love
We pledge to preserve the integrity of our friendship
As we face each new day rising to seize its promise together.

To symbolize our commitment
We exchange these rings
Three intertwining circles to represent
Past, present, and future
To remind us that the past informs the present
And the present shapes the future.

And from this continuity that we experience together
We know with certainty
That our lives are intertwined
Beyond the passing importance of this ritual
To create the bond that is family.

We exchanged our rings and kissed and bowed to the applause that filled
the room. I felt so gratified to have done this in the company of people we
loved. After dinner a lively and raucous women's band played. Everybody
danced, men with men, women with women, men and women together.
Between dances guests stepped up to an open microphone and, in a self-

indulgence that we thoroughly enjoyed, paid tribute to us individually and as a couple. It was a memorable evening, photographed, videotaped, and reported in the gay press. One account began: "Marlene Deitrich would not have been out of place, nor would the ghost of Tyrone Power have disturbed the atmosphere by so much as a ripple. That is, not if Power had dragged Errol Flynn from his sepulchral closet and Deitrich had shown up with Garbo on her arm."

Our recommitment at fifteen years remains a cardinal event in our shared history. We did it to rejoice in our union and to mark the passage of our time together. I heartily recommend the experience whether it's done elaborately with a cast of hundreds or simply with a few family and friends. It is about paying tribute to the viability of these partnerships that are so often trivialized or maligned. We need to show the world, and not incidentally the gay and lesbian part of it as well, that couples can have the long life together so many seek to have.

Today Terry and I are approaching our twenty-ninth anniversary and planning another celebration. Many of those who came to our fifteenth are no longer with us, but we will dance in their honor, remembering them, feeling them among us, and loving them. We will acknowledge where we have been and where we are now, but most of all we will celebrate our incredible good luck at being who we are.

In the late 1980s I had occasion to visit Stanford University, the school from which I had fled decades earlier because it seemed unthinkable to me to be homosexual on that hallowed ground. Walking around the campus, I was startled to come upon a huge banner stretched across the front of the Old Firehouse: GAY PEOPLE'S UNION. When I got back to Los Angeles, I called Stanford to ask about the Gay People's Union. I got a very pleasant young man who explained that the Gay People's Union has been succeeded by a few other organizations: the Gay and Lesbian Alliance, the Lesbian and Gay and Bisexual Community Center, the Stanford Organization for Lesbian and Gay Equality, the Gay and Lesbian Peer Counseling Group, the Stanford Gay and Lesbian Faculty and Staff Network, the Lesbian, Gay, and Bisexual Speakers Bureau, the Stanford Gay and Lesbian Alumni Club, and gay and lesbian student associations within the Schools of Law, Medicine, Business, and Education. By the time he got through this list I was shaking my head in wonder, remembering the isolation I'd felt at Stanford, the shame and embarrassment about being homosexual. I'd had to leave college to pursue being gay. Now young people go to college to do that. I felt thankful I'd lived long enough to witness this incredible sea change.

In 1992 my relationship with Stanford came full circle. I was asked to present the keynote speech for Stanford's Gay and Lesbian Pride Week. Forty-four years later, I was back, but this time not the frightened victim, undefended against my own and others' homophobia, desperately running away from myself. I was a proud activist, representing the strength that a positive gay identity enables. I told the story of Janet's seduction scene, which brought giggles from the audience, and I recounted my flight from Stanford, which brought silence—disbelief, sadness, or perhaps just an inability to comprehend what that experience would have been like. Speaking to those students was healing for me, a reinforcement of my faith in the future and a reminder that the gay and lesbian movement will continue to grow, gain momentum, be unstoppable. It already is.

April 1993, we are back for another March on Washington, this time with one million participants, according to march officials, less than half that number according to U.S. Park Police, as usual underestimating the crowd. In any case, there were a lot of people, and it took more than six hours for the march to be completed. There were the usual Christian counter-demonstrators along the route, the NoMoHomos crowd, as we called them, screaming through bullhorns for us to "repent," waving their absurd antigay signs, heckling, being mostly ignored or laughed at by the marchers.

The rally following the march was a mixed bag of stirring speeches and some runaway comic performers who caused me, and many others, to wince at their crudity. Nongay politicians and celebrities added their voices to ours in the plea for an end to antigay discrimination, and gay leaders spoke to the issues of equality, access, and empowerment for the gay and lesbian citizens of the United States. A high-visibility theme at the 1993 march was gays in the military, and many gay and lesbian veterans marched in uniform to highlight the controversy raging over lifting the ban on gays and lesbians serving openly in the military. As in 1987, there was another mass wedding ceremony outside the Internal Revenue Service Building, and the quilt panels added since the last march were laid out in the early morning while the names of many of the thousands who had died since 1987 were slowly read.

There were also wonderful social occasions. Marvin Liebman gave a party

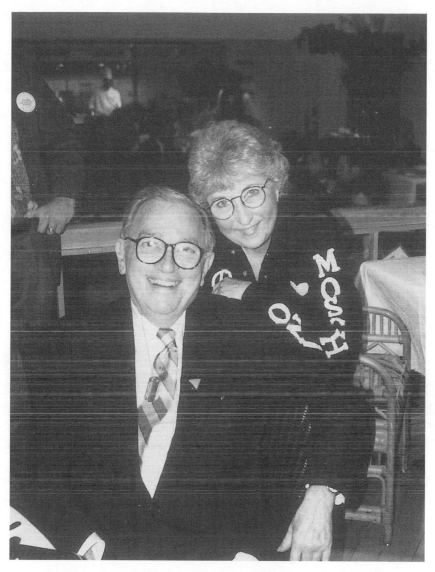

With Marvin Liebman at a dinner in Washington, D.C., the night before
the 1993 march.

on Saturday afternoon that was like a class reunion of the entire gay rights
movement. I met Larry Kramer for the first time and learned the well-kept
secret that he is not the raging bull he often comes off as in the media, but
a sweet, gentle, affable man. Of course the next afternoon, as his voice blared
across the rally site from the stage, angrily castigating Bill "the Welsher"

Clinton and Donna "Do Nothing" Shalala, the sweet, gentle image turned back into that of the more familiar Larry Kramer, hell-raiser.

The night before the march, Richard Rouilard took over one of Washington's newest upscale restaurants for an elegant dinner party, offering a brief respite from the pain of the quilt, the joy of the wedding, and the anticipation of the monumental undertaking of the next day, many hundreds of thousands of gay and lesbian people marching through the streets of Washington to show ourselves to the world.

Comments printed in the *Los Angeles Times* the day after the March surely typified the good news/bad news reaction of many straight onlookers to the scene. "I'm scared," admitted a woman from Baltimore as she stood with her husband watching the chanting, smiling gays and lesbians stream by hour after hour. "I didn't realize there were so many. It scares me to see so many of them. . . . It's unbelievable to see how much they've organized."

Los Angeles, 1989. I was enjoying the party so much, I didn't want to leave. Gay writers and editors from New York were in town for the first Words Project for AIDS awards dinner the next night. The talk was of books, and publishing-world gossip. I loved it and I wanted more. How to do that? I hadn't organized anything for years, but I immediately set about forming plans to start a Los Angeles group for gay and lesbian writers. I invited two friends to lunch, Mark Thompson, author and former senior editor at the *Advocate,* and Jim Spada, who wrote celebrity biographies. They welcomed the idea of a writers' group, and we developed a list of local people to invite. The Los Angeles Gay and Lesbian Writers' Circle was born at that lunch.

Starting in July 1989, the Circle met monthly, with founding members Thompson, Spada, myself, and other Los Angeles writers: Paul Monette, Bernard Cooper, Michael Nava, Michael Lassell, Katherine Forrest, Larry Duplechan, Malcolm Boyd, Eric Latzky, and Barry Sandler (who wrote the early gay-themed feature film *Making Love*). Each month we read from our works-in-progress, commenting on one another's manuscripts, often getting a first view of books that would soon appear on booksellers' shelves. And, as always, there was the gossip about writers, publishers, editors, and agents. It was a fun, exciting group, and I looked forward with great anticipation to every meeting.

I read often from the first version of this memoir. One member of the group who was particularly attentive to my readings was Paul Monette, who announced at one point that listening to me had inspired him to write his own autobiography. Soon he was reading from the manuscript that would appear as *Becoming a Man*. I was still struggling with the writing of my book when *Becoming a Man* was published and won the National Book Award, an honor everyone in our writer's group took personally, especially me.

Reading Paul's book I immediately saw what was missing in mine. I wrote to him:

> It is really a powerful book. I finished it yesterday and I am still reso-
> nating to it. You said I inspired you to write an autobiography. Well,
> now you have inspired me to rewrite mine, differently (if I can), to
> get down in my guts and dig out some of those feelings I have so
> efficiently neutralized over the years. . . . Writing an autobiography is
> like therapy in that neither one works if it's just about telling stories.
> As therapists we sometimes get lazy and just listen to the client's stories,
> especially if they are juicy, but we all know better. The story is just the
> top layer and you have to get down below to really know and help the
> person. I think I've been afraid to be known in so intimate a way so
> I've just tried to make my stories as amusing and interesting as possi-
> ble. From reading your book I see that it's the pain and the passion
> that makes it all come to life. Whether it's anger, or despair, or love,
> or lust, it's the raw feeling that helps the reader tap into his/her own
> emotionality and know there is a commonality to experience that binds
> us all together. You have been very courageous in letting yourself be
> known in a core way. I am going to try to do that too though I doubt
> I will succeed in blasting through decades of defenses sufficiently to
> be able to let the cry out as compellingly as you have. But, I'm going
> to try, and that is your gift to me.

The Los Angeles Gay and Lesbian Writers' Circle lasted about two years. After that time attendance by the original members began to wane as people moved out of town, went on tours, or coped with illness. With the influx of new members, mostly young people who had never been published, the ambience of the group changed. There was less of the old-pro publishing gossip and more of the kinds of questions that new young writers have about how to *get* published. The group did go on for a while but eventually faded away, although many from the original group remained friends and stayed in touch.

The biggest bonus of the Writers' Circle for me was the close friendship that evolved from it with Paul Monette. I had known Paul for twenty years and often saw him at social events, but we were just acquaintances. His first lover, Roger Horowitz, was Sheldon Andelson's half brother, and where Sheldon went, Paul and Roger were usually to be found. In those days Paul was a different person. He was aloof, often writing poems (or something) in his ever-present notebook, too stoned, I concluded, to be available for serious conversation. More than once, I'd seen him pull out a joint and smoke it at a public event.

When Roger died in the late 1980s, Paul began writing about AIDS and a startling transformation occurred in him. He was a man on fire, writing from his gut with a poet's understanding of how words can transcend their own meanings. His book about Roger's illness and death, *Borrowed Time,* was a crossover success, bringing to many nongay readers their first understanding of what AIDS was all about.

As I came to know Paul in the Writers' Circle he was anything but aloof. He was emotionally available, incredibly present, and a joy to be with. At first, it was the sheer pleasure of his intelligence and wit that made being with him so enjoyable. Later, as he became ill with AIDS himself, I was inspired by his courage in dealing with the virus's incredible assaults on his body. I thought about my own experiences with illness and the ease with which I'd often allowed the invader to take over and debilitate my spirit as well as my body. I vowed that in future I would try to follow Paul's example. He fought for every minute of normalcy he could command in the context of a life taken over by drugs and doctors and endless infusions. His partner, Winston Wilde, took very good care of him and supported his insistence on keeping up contacts with the family of friends who loved him.

In 1994 Paul was beginning to have the emaciated, haunted look of a person in the end stage of AIDS, but incredibly he was still traveling, going on cruises with his field hospital of IV equipment and medications, going out to dinner, seeing movies, appearing on television, being interviewed by the press. But in November, Paul began talking about "just being done with it." When he told me this, it took me a few minutes to realize he meant done with his life. The side effects of the medications were too enervating. He'd had enough. He asked me what I thought about that. I told him I would respect whatever he decided. He said he wanted to keep talking to me about it. I dearly hoped I would have the wisdom to say the right things to him.

Around mid-December Paul made his decision. He stopped most of his

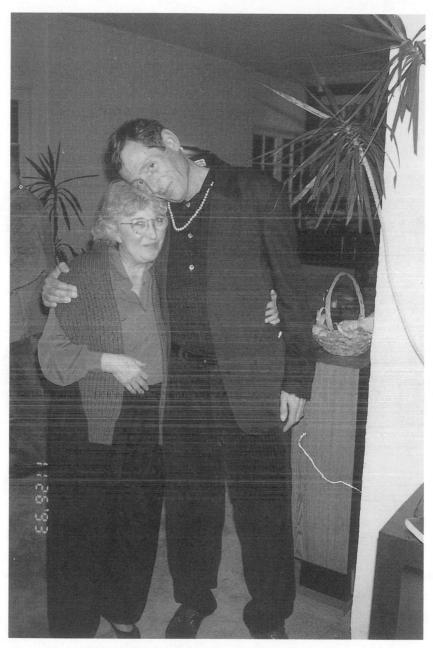

Paul Monette in 1993, already sick but very much out and about.

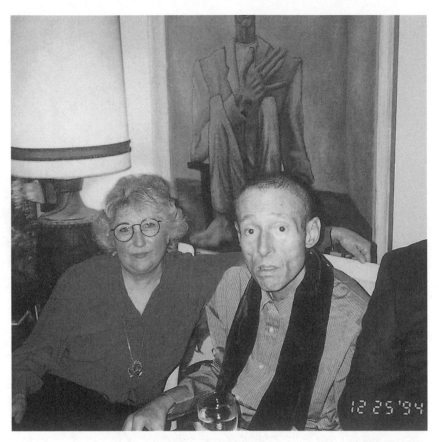
Paul Monette in 1994, spending his last Christmas at a party at our house.

treatments and medical appointments. I'd been in New York, and on my return he apologized for making this decision without me. That startled me. I hadn't realized I'd become that important to him. I knew what he meant to me on so many different levels, but I had not admitted to consciousness the depth of the affection he might be feeling toward me. I was very moved. To give Winston some respite, and to spend more time with Paul, I began making dinner at their house. Paul liked pasta, one food he was able to eat, so I cooked spaghetti. Shuffling in his slow gait, Paul would follow me around his kitchen telling me where everything was, although I'd been there before and knew perfectly well where everything was. He started calling me "Spaghetti Betty."

"Hello, Spaghetti Betty. How about making some dinner for me tonight?"

When the holidays came we knew it would be Paul's last Christmas, so

Terry and I gave a large party on Christmas Eve. We decorated the house to a fare-thee-well to make the party as festive as possible. Paul came with his morphine pump attached to his side. I seated him against a wall with a semicircle of chairs in front of him. He merrily held court as guests took turns conversing with him. Watching Paul, I observed that some people were easier for him to take than others. When the person facing him was carrying on too energetically or too long, Paul's fingers would slip down to the pump and ever so unobtrusively dial it up.

I hovered more than I should have.

"Paul, do you need more water?" "Paul, would you like more Kleenex?" "Paul, would you like a bag for your Kleenex?" "Paul, do you want me to take that plate away?"

Finally realizing I was overdoing it, inundating him with help more for my sake than his, I withdrew, leaving him to his conversations. Paul stayed for hours, talking, laughing, and in his typical fashion, culling every moment of enjoyment out of his last Christmas party.

It's January and I'm talking on the phone to John Rechy, an old friend and the writer of those splendid books in the 1970s that so boldly portrayed gay male life as no writer had done before. John is now a highly respected teacher of writing. He knows I am a friend of Paul's, and he tells me that he's never met Paul and he would give anything to be able to do that. I convey his request to Paul, who says that he would be delighted to meet John. So one Saturday afternoon I take John Rechy to Paul Monette's house in the Hollywood Hills.

Paul had been off his medications for about a month and his mind was crystal clear. He and John formed a mutual admiration society, praising each other for the risks they had each taken in their writing. Although John was shy by nature, he and Paul connected enthusiastically through their war stories about editors, publishers, and especially reviewers. Winston and I remained on the edge of the conversation, as Paul and John fed off one another, ripping into accounts of what were once devastating experiences in the publishing world, now just anecdotes to laugh about. Paul summed up the similarities between the two of them: "We are two who have refused to let them put us in an intellectual closet."

I circle this little group, taking pictures, and as I do I feel the sadness of imagining Paul no longer here. I tell myself there will be time soon enough

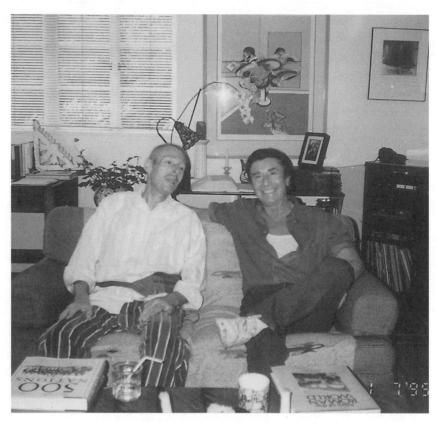

John Rechy with Paul Monette in January 1995. Paul had stopped his treatment
and was feeling good. He died about four weeks later.

for these thoughts, right now I should enjoy the fact that he is here and this
meeting, which I arranged, is taking place. After a while Paul starts to look a
little frayed. John sees it too and begins his good-byes. The two men hug,
mutually agreeing that they are so happy to have met and vowing to talk again.

On January 29, Terry and I are at Paul and Winston's for another "Spaghetti
Betty" special. At the end of the evening Paul stands up to escort us to the
door, always the gentleman. Although he is unable to straighten his body,
bent in half like a very old man, he shuffles behind us to the door. Terry
and I had just lost our best friend, Stan Ziegler, to a sudden, unexpected
death from a non-AIDS-related illness. Paul was acquainted with Stan, who

lived just a block from him and he knew how close we had been. Just as the door is opened, Paul moves closer to us, his voice just above a whisper.

"Now I know Stan's death has been hard on you. Remember, I'm here for emotional support. Call me anytime."

I walk out in a daze, tears filling my eyes. How extraordinary. This man, now less than two weeks away from his own death, is offering himself to us for emotional support. That was essential Paul Monette.

On February 7, a call came from Winston. Paul hadn't eaten in several days, and Winston was sure the end was near; we should come anytime. I went that evening. People gathered in the living room of Paul and Winston's house warned me not to expect Paul to be able to speak. In the bedroom I found him laid out flat in his bed, covers up to his neck, his eyes closed. I told Paul who I was and he nodded. I put my hand over his two hands, one folded over the other and found they were blazing hot. He tried to talk but couldn't. I told him I knew he wanted to talk and how frustrating it must be for him not to be able to, but that it was okay, we'd just sit quietly together. After a while Paul appeared to sleep. I whispered that I was going to talk to Winston. He nodded. I leaned over him and said, "I love you, Paul." He opened his eyes and in a perfectly clear voice answered, "I love you too."

On February 10, Paul died.

18

I'd just returned from Paul's memorial service to find my sister's voice on the answering machine.

"Mom died." Full of feeling about Paul, I somehow couldn't find it in myself to feel anything about my mother's death, except concern that very soon I would have to organize another funeral.

February 1995 was the month of deaths for us. On the 5th, Terry and I put on an elaborate memorial service for our friend Stan Ziegler. On the 10th, Paul died, and on the 19th we said good-bye at his memorial service. On the 26th, yet another funeral, when my mother would be brought back to Los Angeles from Ohio to be interred in our family crypt at Westwood Village Memorial Park.

Following a debilitating heart attack and stroke ten years before, my mother had been living in Wexner-Heritage House in Columbus, Ohio, one of the premier skilled-nursing facilities in the United States. Although she had lived in Los Angeles for many years, her relocation to Ohio seemed a good solution because my sister Stephanie had had a more positive relationship with our mother than I. My sister also had four grown children, some with children of their own, a ready-made crew to visit and care for grandma.

Terry and I paid the nursing home bills and went to Columbus once a year to give my mother a birthday party, actually jolly occasions with family, nursing home staff, and residents in attendance. I was grateful to my sister for taking on the responsibility of caring for our mother and doing a much better job than I could have been able to do, since I had long ago resigned emotionally from much of a relationship with my mother.

Relatives came for the funeral from far and wide. We had a simple cryptside service in this tiny cemetery so famous as the final resting place of celebrities that tourists from all over the world visit it. My father attended the funeral with his wife, Trude. When my mother's casket was being angled into the crypt, my father began to wail.

"That's Eve in there. Let me say good-bye again!"

It took a while for me to calm him down as everyone sat in silence. I chose to forgo reminding my father that he had been divorced from my mother for forty-five years and had had five other wives since her. Was he upset because she had been the mother of his children? No, I think it was about one more experience of letting go of life, which he knew he was in the process of doing himself.

Following the funeral ceremony, relatives trekked around the cemetery oohing and aahing over the familiar names on the graves and crypts—Marilyn Monroe, Natalie Wood, Donna Reed, Daryl Zanuck, Truman Capote, Buddy Rich, Burt Lancaster, Will Durant, John Cassavetes, Armand Hammer, and on and on. Auspicious company to be in, folks whom Terry and I will someday join in our little corner of Westwood Village Memorial Park's "Sanctuary of Serenity."

It was disconcerting when my father went from walking with a cane to using a walker. When they brought the wheelchair in, it was clear that he was losing his ability, and perhaps his will, to be self-sustaining at all. At eighty-nine, he had slipped into a kind of twilight of awareness, reality coming and going. Debilitated by age and dementia, he was being cared for in an assisted-living facility, where he mostly sat in his recliner chair, completely dressed every day, hat and all, waiting for the next adventure of his life to begin. He looked good and was glad to see anyone who came to visit, although he usually didn't remember who they were to begin with and forgot they had been there two minutes after they left.

There can be a lot unnerving about the kind of role reversal that occurs when the child becomes the caretaker of the parent. Watching my aging parents decline and become helpless was disorienting, and I was not prepared for it. I don't know what I expected, but when Trude could no longer take care of my father and moved to Florida to live with her daughter, I became his sole caretaker, ready or not.

I never felt either of my parents took very good care of me, but the issue was moot when I was faced with the reality of a frail and fragile old man, helpless, needy, and depending on me. If there is any small part of a person that has not yet grown up, no matter what their age, parenting a parent will expedite the process. Fortunately for me, I have a partner who took a major role in caring for my father. She lightened the load enough to keep me sane, at least most of the time. I am not a good hands-on person in this caretaking business. I'm terrific at organizing, planning, and arranging, but not at direct care. I tend to become confounded about where I stop and the other person begins. Contact with my father's confusion and panic triggered the same feelings in me. I often had to remind myself that what was happening to him was not happening to me.

If I thought I was not ready for the responsibility of being a caretaker to my father, I discovered I was even less prepared when he developed an infection and high fever that destroyed the last vestige of cognition he was ever to enjoy.

Bearing witness to the disturbing climax of my father's life, I felt rage once again at the forces that hold hostage the kinds of change that could enhance our humanity. In the name of religious belief, conservatives deny other people the dignity of an assisted release from the torment of physical pain or the blackout of a life already surrendered to death. How lucky our dogs and cats are that religious conservatives haven't invaded the realms of their lives so they can still be afforded the dignified death that is denied so many unfortunate human beings. I don't think I have time for another activist cause now, but this is one that strikes at the heart when it becomes personally relevant.

The phone call came at 4:30 A.M. "Your father has died." It was over, and I was relieved, for him and for me. Then there was the myriad of tasks that always follow a death—the calls to relatives, the arrangements at the cemetery, the disposition of belongings, the planning of the funeral. I could handle all that, my feelings muted, no deep grief to cloud the brain. My father as I'd known him had been gone a long time already.

The funeral attracted more people than I thought it would—cousins, a few of my father's surviving friends, my stepmother's grown grandchildren to whom my father had been the only grandfather they had ever known, and Carol, the widow of Trude's son, Paul. Friends of ours came, which touched me realizing how true a family friends become in the gay and lesbian world. My sister, Stephanie, and her daughter, Dina, had spent the last six days of my father's life with him and had already gone back to Ohio. Trude had just suffered a heart attack in Florida and was not allowed to travel to the funeral, much to her distress.

Eulogies were delivered by cousins, Carol, and step-grandchildren. They were mostly in the same vein, what a high flyer my father was and how he had shown them all extravagant good times, at the racetrack and at pricey restaurants and country clubs. As I listened, I had to work not to feel resentful thinking of the times he had gone back on his promises to help me financially earlier in my life, of the last ten years when Terry and I had sacrificed to support him because by then he was dead broke. All of his high flying had been without a net.

As is so often true at these closing ceremonies, the idealized person is center stage, as it should be, but I could not resist one tweak when it was my turn to say a few words.

"My father's life was a pleasure palace in which he was the main inhabitant."

Terry glared at me, arms crossed, warning me with her eyes not to go any further along this path. I knew I shouldn't, and didn't, my dedication to honesty and reality giving way to the exigencies of protocol. Our lesbian rabbi, Denise Eger, presided over the religious part of the service as she had done at my mother's funeral, adding the properly serious note that the occasion deserved.

The Kaddish completed, everyone sat silently, waiting, a slight breeze ruffling the flowers that surrounded the coffin. I stepped to the podium, thanked those present for coming, and invited them all to join us for lunch. People began to move in slow motion, coming to me and to Terry, murmuring words of condolence, hugging us. I sleepwalked through the luncheon and was glad to get home to begin the letting go and my adjustment to the new freedom of never having to worry again about another emergency phone call to attend to my father. Cousins-in-the-know complimented me on taking such good care of my father, given his behavior toward me through much of my life. It had never occurred to me that I had a choice in the matter.

"You people are disgusting and repulsive."

"Why don't you get on your broom and fly off somewhere."

"Homosexuality is a negation of life!"

"God hates you!"

When the expanded edition of *Positively Gay* came out in 1992, I appeared on thirteen radio talk shows. Those radio shows proved to be a very wild ride because President Clinton, early in his administration, had just announced his intent to lift the ban on gays in the military. The homophobes smelled blood and fell upon their phones.

While I was trying to talk about being "positively gay," the callers were telling me that I was an abomination to God, and the United States would become defenseless if homosexual perverts were allowed in the military. They read to me from the Bible, asked why gays wanted to destroy the family, and protested having our sinful "lifestyle" shoved down their throats. One man wanted to talk to me about homosexual cockroaches, which he absolutely knew for a fact existed, and another announced he was going to show me what he thought of me, then emitted a long, lusty belch. I fielded some legitimate queries about why gays do what we do, but even then the tone was hostile. The hosts of these programs were often more outrageous than the callers. I was rattled. Had I been living in a cocoon these last few years? I was shocked at the vitriol, momentarily lost to the ability to respond in any way that made sense, but I had to do something.

Since all of these interviews occurred by phone, from home, I began recording and playing back every program, each time honing my comments until they were concise, and punched home my message, no matter what off-the-wall rant or gastrointestinal eruptions I was confronted with. When I finished, I had the beginnings of a book on how to deal with people in homophobic encounters. Of course, most gay and lesbian people would never have to cope with the kinds of irrational raving I experienced in these talk-show experiences, but the same underlying misguided thinking and bigotry is often operative in relationships that have a rational, even caring basis.

In 1996, *Setting Them Straight: You Can Do Something about Bigotry and Homophobia in Your Life,* was published. I tried in this book to help gay and lesbian readers overcome the fear we have all had when it comes to speaking up and countering antigay remarks, whether they come from professional homophobes or from someone who is well-intentioned but doesn't know any better. I wrote about what to do in homophobic encounters with family, friends, acquaintances, and strangers and how to cope with such experiences in the workplace. I encouraged anger at injustice and spelled out strategies for managing that anger so it can be used to enable action and accomplish a purpose. Because I believe that we always respond better when we know what makes our opponents tick, I included explanations on why people hate, the nature and origins of prejudice, the purpose of scapegoating, and how to respond to specific comments and questions about being gay or lesbian.

On the book tour for *Setting Them Straight,* I listened to the anguish so many gay and lesbian people felt over antigay attitudes in their families, on the job, and in society in general. I felt like a missionary, encouraging people to get involved in a level of activism they may have never before considered for themselves:

It starts with you being a hero in your own life, overcoming fear, speaking up, going against tradition, breaking the rules, demanding respect. Only you can break the conspiracy of silence in your family, only you can counter bigotry and homophobia in your own life.

It is unusual to have two books published in the same year, but that is what happened to me in 1996. *The Intimacy Dance: A Guide to Long-Term Success in Gay and Lesbian Relationships* was a sequel to *Permanent Partners*. Focusing on the long-term issues inherent in relationships, I was able to draw on my work with over a thousand couples and my own twenty-year partnership.

"I don't understand it. We were so close and suddenly we were so far apart." "We were fighting, but I couldn't stand being angry at her anymore." "I don't know why we go back and forth. It doesn't make sense."

Listening to statements like these from my clients I began to formulate the idea that partners tend, rather routinely, to do a "dance"—moving toward and away from one another as a way of managing the emotional distance between them. The emotional distance between partners is about the level of intimacy between them. Many people need to control how much intimacy they can tolerate at a given time. My hope was to help people better understand their "intimacy dances" since the moves they make are often not even conscious, and therefore mysterious.

In the fall of 1996 I went on my second book tour of the year. Relationship books always generate a lot of interest and I drew large crowds. That not only made me feel good but planted the seeds of a dangerous illusion. I began to think of myself as a guru dispensing wisdom to my adoring public. The folly of that illusion was quickly dispelled when the tour was over and I returned to the isolation of sitting alone at a computer, writing again, faced only with myself and the intimidation of the blank page. This is the crazy process that most writers go through: a year or more of isolation, then the months-long disappearance of the manuscript into the publisher's black hole to be edited and produced, followed by what seems like the overnight bursting forth of a published book (that by then you almost forgot you wrote), and (if you are lucky) the tour that takes you busily from city to city as you

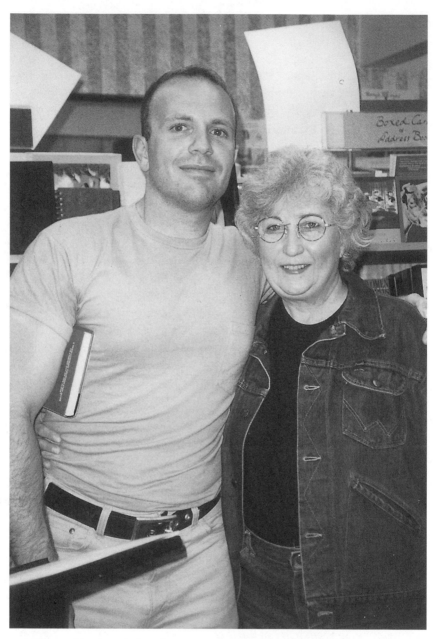

With my friend Michelangelo Signorile who had just read at A Different Light Bookstore in Los Angeles from his book *Outing Yourself,* for which I wrote the foreword. (Courtesy of Edgar B. Anderson)

face the audiences that will very soon disappear to leave you sitting in lonely isolation, writing once again.

One thing that has helped in putting the writing life in perspective is being close to other writers. Friendships with authors like Gabriel Rotello, Michelangelo Signorile, and Felice Picano, among others, provide company in the dilemmas that most professional writers share. My life has been immeasurably enriched by these friendships.

Terry cringed as the *Times* hit the driveway. "I don't want to see it," she said pulling the covers over her head. I went out and picked up the paper. The article began, "Recent allegations of sexual misconduct leveled against the staff of an agency that operates group homes for gay teenagers . . ."

When two people have lived together in an intimate partnership for more than two decades as Terry and I have, what is happening to one is also happening to the other. My cancer surgery was not only my experience, it was also Terry's. When the State of California Department of Social Services began a campaign to discredit Terry's advocacy for gay, lesbian, and transgendered teenagers, to humiliate her and harass her out of the field, it was happening to me too.

"Don't take me away from my home!"

"These are the only people who understand me!"

"This is the only place I have felt safe!"

"I'm not fucking going with you!"

These were the cries of the children of GLASS as they were forcibly removed in a late-night surprise raid on the five GLASS group homes where they lived, removed "for their own protection" because accusations of sexual abuse of these kids had been made against male staff and volunteers. Now these teenagers were being transferred from their gay-affirming environment to juvenile institutions known to be homophobic. Some ran away to the streets, from which they were rescued by GLASS in the first place, one tried to commit suicide.

March 15, 1996, the nightmare began for us when the State of California opened an investigation and assigned an investigator whose agenda was clear: to prove that the allegations against Terry and GLASS staff were true, whether they were or not. In this field, such investigators are called "validators." They do not seek the truth, only evidence to validate what they already believe. Making matters worse was an out lesbian reporter on the *Los Angeles*

Times about whom it was said by her colleagues that she would not be caught dead "pandering" to the gay community. She wrote three articles favoring the state's case, spelling out the accusations in detail, as though she were writing not about allegations but about actual occurrences.

Support for Terry quickly organized all over the country. People who knew her only by reputation called, wrote, faxed, and e-mailed to say that they saw through the allegations and what the state was doing to GLASS. The wagons were circled. People signed newspaper ads supporting Terry and GLASS. We were gratified to have this support, which made it all the more startling that the most notable holdout was the head of the largest gay organization in Los Angeles. Her response was that she must wait to see the outcome of the case before she could be supportive and lend her name. She apparently had no clue that by withholding her support she was abdicating the responsibility of a leader to rise above the fears our opponents work so hard to instill in us. She became a willing conspirator in the state's homophobic witch hunt against GLASS.

Lawyers began the slow process of building a defense against the specific allegations. The most frightening part of all this was the unbridled power of the state to act repeatedly without due process of law and without concern for the terrible toll they exacted on the lives of everyone involved. Nearly a hundred GLASS employees lost their jobs. Kids were displaced. GLASS volunteers were publicly humiliated, their employers advised that they were accused child molesters, their careers halted, legal fees incurred—and all this before there was any day in court, any evidence of wrongdoing. It was a campaign of harassment, the subtext of which was that teenagers who openly identify themselves as gay or lesbian or even questioning should not be cared for in a gay-affirming environment.

The accusation that Terry would condone sexual abuse of GLASS kids by staff, volunteers, and board members was ludicrous. She teaches and trains social workers and child-care workers, has an impeccable reputation of more than thirty years of work with young people, has spent sixteen years building GLASS against many odds. In addition, she is the product of seventeen years of Catholic school and one of the most prudish people I know.

Terry was hurt, depressed, and discouraged, but she was also mobilized, fighting mad, and on top of her game. I was awed by her ability to withstand the humiliation, the blows that came from the *Times* articles, the threats by the state to revoke her license and ban her for life from working in her profession in California.

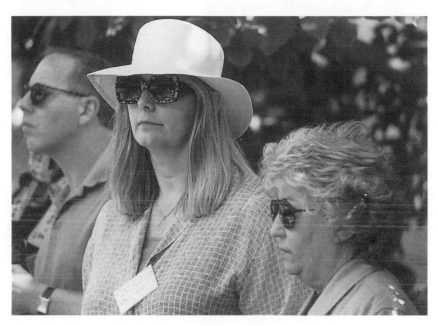

Terry and me . . . still.

I had my own bouts with despair, too. I have a tendency to catastrophize situations, but Terry reminded me that we were not just waiting for the next shoe to drop, we were fighting every day, legally and politically, and we were not going to give up. The GLASS board of directors stood solidly behind Terry, backing her with the necessary funds to do battle in the courts.

Since that terrible day in March 1996, only two cases were ever brought to court. One was dismissed outright, the other had a finding of no sexual misconduct. To avoid a months-long trial that would have bankrupted GLASS, Terry swallowed hard and reluctantly settled with the state, admitting to unspecified wrongdoing and accepting humiliating restrictions on her ability to function in her job. GLASS was put on probation for five years, during which Terry was not allowed to be alone with GLASS kids without another adult present, a restriction designed primarily to humiliate her, since she was never accused of sexual misconduct herself.

For the term of the probation, Terry could not train GLASS child-care workers, a bizarre irony considering she continued to be an official trainer for the children's services workers hired by Los Angeles County. However, accepting the punitive conditions of this compromise enabled GLASS to re-open and do business again. After the settlement GLASS rebuilt. The houses filled with kids again and new projects and programs began. Terry returned to work at her office, and GLASS continues to fulfill its mission, having survived an exhausting, expensive, harrowing attack.

There are important lessons in this story. First is the personal story about what happens in a partnership that is stressed to its limits. One or the other partner may feel so much despair at a given moment that it spills over to affect the other. On days when the state or the press struck particularly painful blows, I panicked and my anxiety did spill out all over the place. But what I came to see was how my self-indulgence only increased Terry's stress, overloading the system, and making it more difficult for either of us to cope. This doesn't mean that being discouraged and frightened shouldn't be talked about; it does mean that when those feelings are expressed, it should be done with a sensitivity to how the level of emotionality is affecting the other person. Several people asked me if the crisis drove us apart. Our relationship only became stronger during the crisis.

There is also a lesson in this story for gay and lesbian rights activism. We must never let our guard down. We must continue to mobilize on every front—political, legal, public education, the media, and in our own lives. We must allow anger against injustice—controlled, directed, and acted upon. We must also take special care to get at the truth of all assaults against us and be ready and willing to extend support when it is needed. We owe that to one another. We owe that to ourselves.

19

The phone call from Washington, D.C., came on a Monday, March 31, 1997. "We've lost Marvin."

It was Chris Bull, the *Advocate* reporter and one of the group of bright young men whom Marvin Liebman kept around him. Devoted, fascinated by his stories, true affection flowing both ways, they were part of Marvin's chosen family.

At first I thought he meant that Marvin had wandered off into the night. "Lost Marvin? When did you see him last?"

"This morning, he died," Chris answered.

"My god, what happened?"

Chris explained that Marvin was having a heart problem Saturday night and went to the hospital. Sunday he rallied enough to be flirting with the male nurses. Everyone thought he was okay, but Sunday night he took a turn for the worse. Five of his friends stayed with him through the night, until he died the next morning. Chris said that the hospital staff didn't know what to make of all these young men—so many grandsons!

It took a while for the news to sink in. Marvin dead? I'd had the feeling that he would always be around, always be part of my world. "Don't be ridiculous, darling," he said. "We'll be friends the rest of our lives." He was right, we were friends the rest of his life.

In 1989 I called Marvin to say that I was writing about him and that boy, Leon, he had picked up in Cannes and shipped back to New York in 1963. I said, "I guess I can't write that, can I? You're still in the closet."

"Oh, darling, go ahead. Who cares anymore," Marvin blurted out. "It's time I came out anyway!" And that was the beginning of Marvin Liebman's rocket launch into gay celebrity at age sixty-seven. He decided to come out in a big way, by writing a letter to his close friend Bill Buckley to be published in Buckley's *National Review*. In the process of writing that letter, Marvin asked me to find some antigay comments from conservatives that he could quote. I called my friend Mark Thompson, then a senior editor at the *Advocate* and told him the story.

"What!?" Mark said. "Listen, I'll call you right back!"

When Mark called back it was to say that the *Advocate* was going to do a story on Marvin and put him on the cover—Prominent Conservative Comes Out! Marvin was thrilled and immediately threw himself into it. There were talk-show appearances, the lecture circuit, a syndicated column in the gay press, and fame as the former strategist for the American conservative movement turned gay rights activist! He told the story of his life in a book, *Coming Out Conservative.*

I became Marvin's mentor, introducing him to the players, the backstage scene, and the dynamics of the contemporary gay movement. I took delight in that because early in our relationship I was often tongue-tied when it came to discussing politics with him because he was the political professional and I was just a naive bleeding-heart liberal. Now the tables were turned.

"Darling, do I have to say gay *and* lesbian every time?" he'd plead.

For a long time he sent me his syndicated columns to edit, and I kept him politically correct until he caught on and didn't need my mentoring any more.

Marvin was a great talker. He liked to stay in touch, keep the connection, calling me so often that in recent years I had sometimes felt annoyed when I heard him on the other end of the line. Now I'd like to feel annoyed again. I miss that raspy voice and his usual opening: "Darling, it's Marvin. Can you talk?"

"Go without hate but not without rage. Heal the world," Paul Monette proclaimed in a speech accepting one of his honorary doctorates.

We can't heal the whole world but we can certainly work to relieve the pain of alienation that ignorance and prejudice cause to many with whom we share this planet. In my own corner of the world I have tried to be that kind of healer. Recently, I've decided to go one step further, to design a future for gay and lesbian people that elevates our status from a group discriminated against to a constituency wielding the voting power and the political influence our numbers make possible. The future I'm predicting is described in the novel I have begun to write about gay life in the late twenty-first century.

According to my vision of things to come, the road from the present will be a rocky one. Trauma, conflict, and fragmentation will precede reorganization and harmony in the new gay and lesbian reality. Predicting the future is a dicey business. Redesigning society is a leap off the precipice. I've chosen to take that leap, and while it may be heart-stopping at times, it is ultimately magical to experience the freedom of invention.

So I spend my time these days anticipating the coming decades and trying to stay one step ahead of the changes already underway. Among other things, writing about the future has eased my passage into the new century, something that I've looked forward to with apprehension (will I make it?) and regard with disbelief now that it's here (have I really been alive this long?).

In this memoir I have traveled back to the past to search for an understanding of how I got to be who I am. The trip has been at times frustrating and confusing. My life has been such a crazy quilt of identities, some formed out of adolescent dreams, some out of what I thought other people wanted me to be, and some out of circumstances of fate that forced definitions upon me. Now I believe I have finally arrived at an identity that is generated from the inside, integrating external influences and my own strong sense of who and what I am.

As I look back over the arc of my life, I see the fragments that I must piece together and organize into a meaningful whole. But I had to start with the fragments, the scenes that flash across the screen, to reconstruct past reality. Sometimes I have trouble reconciling the different images of myself that pop into view. Which one was really me?

Was that actually me in the 1950s in a locked psychiatric ward under suicide watch, wrists tethered to the bed, too confused to understand what had happened to me? Or was that me the following year, working on the staff of that same hospital, white coat, keys to the kingdom jangling in my pocket, a psychiatric aide leading others around the landscape that had once confined me?

Was that me in the 1960s traveling the growth center circuit conducting workshops called the Quest for Love, so determined to be heterosexual that Michael Murphy called me "the bunny girl of the Human Potential Movement"? Or was that me in the 1970s marching in gay pride parades, reborn as an activist, on the lecture circuit speaking for and about the gay and lesbian community, creating organizations, convinced that I could change the world since I had so amazingly changed myself?

Perhaps it was the real me in the 1980s shutting out all distractions to concentrate on being a homebody, steeped in domesticity and the demands of building a loving relationship? Or was the real me that person in the 1990s, touring the country, being interviewed, enjoying the attention of bookstore audiences, fans telling me that my books have changed their lives?

Maybe there are no contradictions in this mosaic, only a progression from one stage of life to another. We move on, but we retain the stories that give shape and texture to our narrative, that hold the clues to how we have become who we are. I have searched my stories in an effort to connect the dots and come at last to the final outline of identity. I set out on this trail with some trepidation. I wasn't sure what I would find in traveling back to these beginnings—embarrassment, sadness, regret, amusement, or elation that it's almost over and I've survived. I found all these things.

I have tried in this book to echo the sentiments I've heard so often from the people I've worked with over the years and to say, "I too am flawed." "I too have wondered if I'm loved." "I too have despaired."

But I have also studied myself and sought new possibilities for my life. I've tried harder to allow love, to believe in my own competence, to trust the inner cues that tell me what I need and want. Most unexpected of all was the discovery that being different has given my life meaning and potency, that I never again have to hide who I am, in any way, from anyone.

Life for me at the beginning of this new century is a season of grace. As I write this, the dogs are asleep in the patches of sunlight that filter into the living room through the French doors. Terry is in the next room clicking away on her computer. The rest of the house is quiet. Everything is in order.

LIVING OUT

Gay and Lesbian Autobiographies

Joan Larkin and David Bergman
General Editors